medical readings
on
first aid

oliver e. byrd, stanford university

thomas r. byrd, de anza college

boyd & fraser publishing company
san francisco, california

This book is in the
BOYD & FRASER MEDICAL READINGS SERIES
Copyright © 1971 by Boyd & Fraser Publishing Company. All rights reserved.
No part of this work may be reproduced or used in any form or by any means—
graphic, electronic, or mechanical, including photo-copying, recording,
taping, or information and retrieval systems—without written permission
from the publisher. Manufactured in the United States of America.
Library of Congress Catalog Card Number: 72-152746
ISBN: 0-87835-019-5

1 2 3 . 3 2 1

preface

The American National Red Cross with its outstanding contributions for more than 50 years to the preparation and training of first aid instructors has been the inspiration for the production of this book. The editors have received encouragement in its preparation from officers of the Palo Alto Chapter and the Western Regional Office in San Francisco.

The undersigned have long felt that the standard textbook and the instructor's manual should be supplemented by a third-level book to give deeper understandings to instructors and college students who enroll in first aid courses. Other uses are visualized for a medical readings book on first aid for pre-nursing and nursing groups, pre-medical students, and a large number of students in paramedical fields.

There are more than 7,000 medical journals published on a regular basis throughout the world. The editors have access to about 5,000. Most of them are found only in medical libraries and are generally unavailable to students of first aid and their instructors, even though they constitute a vast treasure chest of knowledge on emergency conditions.

The medical readings of this book have been screened, selected, condensed and simplified over a quarter of a century by the editors. They represent a very small sample of the medical research and experience contained in the total medical publications of 25 years. Nevertheless, the editors believe that these readings will begin the process of deepening the understanding and improving the competence of first aid instructors and practitioners.

Most of the readings were not chosen for their first aid content alone. Most were selected because they would provide information over and beyond the provision of emergency care so that better comprehensions and broadened understandings would qualify the first aid instructor for better responses to student inquiries and thus improve discussions of first aid problems.

Some of the inclusions have appeared in previous publications. Permission of the Stanford University Press to use these materials is gratefully acknowledged.

T.R.B.
O.E.B.

contents

1   some general principles 1

    the severely injured patient 1
    multiple injuries from accidents 3
    first aid for traffic victims 5
    immediate handling of traffic injuries 7
    removal of persons injured in auto accidents 8
    transportation of accident victims 10
    wound healing 11
    application of cold to injuries 12

2   cardiac emergencies 15

    mobile units for heart attack victims 15
    first aid for heart attacks 16
    external cardiac compression 18
    external cardiac massage 20
    broken ribs from external cardiac massage 21
    cessation of breathing and heart action 22
    sudden death of athletes 23
    causes of disturbances in rhythm of the heart 25

3   cessation of breathing 29

    fundamental mechanisms in breathing 29
    artificial respiration 30
    survival with artificial respiration 32
    the Eve method of artificial respiration 34
    inadequacy of the Schafer method of artificial respiration 36
    foreign bodies in air passages 37
    breath-holding spells in children 38
    tuberculosis from artificial respiration 40

contents

4 drowning 43

drowning 43
some facts about drowning 45
care of the near-drowning victim 48
an analysis of 163 drowning accidents 49

5 bleeding 53

bleeding disorders 53
bleeding in head injury 54
symptoms and signs of brain hemorrhage 56
emergency care of injury to blood vessels 57
proper use of the tourniquet 58
basic mechanisms in nosebleed 61
nosebleed 63

6 shock 65

eight basic causes of shock 65
shock lung 67
shock from diminished blood volume 69
shock and its effects on human cells 70
bee sting and anaphylactic shock 72

7 head injuries 77

head injuries 77
examination of head injuries 79
severe head injuries 81
late complications in head injuries 82
brain damage from deceleration of the automobile 83
brain damage from head injuries 85
concussion in children 87
results of severe head injuries in childhood 88
emergency care of facial injuries 89
injuries to the face 90

contents

        broken nose in childhood   92
        loss of hearing from head injury   93
        broken eardrums in children   93

8   **psychiatric emergencies   95**

        psychiatric symptoms of children   95
        emergency psychotherapy   96
        brief psychotherapy   97
        emotional disorders and traffic accidents   99
        the potential suicide   100
        attempted suicides   102
        attempted suicides in adolescents   103
        delinquency and accidents   104
        psychiatric emergencies in children   105
        child abuse   107

9   **drug reactions   109**

        emergency care for drug reactions   109
        barbiturate overdosage   110
        handling of bad trips   112
        effects of drugs in the body   114
        multiple effects of drugs   115
        near-fatal reaction to heroin   117
        symptoms of heroin usage   118
        heroin overdosage and the lungs   120
        x-ray evidence of heroin intoxication   121
        symptoms of narcotic addiction in the newborn   123

10   **poisonings   125**

        health effects of insecticides   125
        pesticide poisoning in children   127
        immediate treatment of poisoning   128
        poison accidents in childhood   130
        household poisonings   131

contents

aspirin poisoning 134
lead poisoning in children 135
throat damage from corrosives 136

11   internal injuries 139

injuries to the spine 139
injuries to the neck 140
first aid for spinal cord injuries 142
should pregnant women wear seat belts? 143
when the pregnant woman is hurt 144
seat belt injuries 147
blunt injuries to the chest 149
abdominal injuries 150
rupture of the spleen 152
injury to the kidney 152

12   burns 155

burns of children 155
burning clothes 156
cold treatment of burns 157
burns on the face 159
critical results of burns 160
biologic treatment of burns 161

13   electrical injuries 163

electrical burns of the mouth 163
electrical injuries 164
electrical accidents 167
deaths from lightning 169

14   heat injuries 171

fatalities and medical effects of heat and exercise 171
four effects of excessive heat 172

heat stroke 174
salt losses in hot environments 175
265 cases of heat disease 176

15 cold injuries 179

effects of frostbite on growth 179
accidental deaths from cold weather 181
injury from excessive cold 182
the windchill factor 183
frostbite 186
frostbite as a military problem 187
protection of feet immersed in cold water 188

16 bites and stings 189

anaphylactic reactions to stings 189
deaths from stings and bites 190
brown spider bites 192
black widow spider poisoning 193
the black widow spider 195
snakebite 196
facts and fictions about snakebite 198
snakebite 201
animal bites and rabies 204
dog bite 205

17 emergencies of vision 207

visual complications from drugs 207
eye burns and tear gas 208
detachment of the retina 209
foreign bodies in the eye 211
eye injuries 213
alkali burns of the eye 215
eye emergencies in industry 217

contents

18 **dental injuries 219**

    persistent bleeding after tooth extraction 219
    treatment of injured teeth 220
    dental injuries 222

19 **dislocations and joint injuries 225**

    dislocation of the shoulder 225
    shoulder injuries 226
    self-reduction of a dislocated shoulder 228
    soft tissue injuries of the knee 229
    ankle injuries 230

20 **unconsciousness 233**

    fainting 233
    fainting spells 234
    multiple causes of unconsciousness 236
    unconscious diabetic patient 237
    head injuries and coma 240
    coma mechanisms 241
    unconsciousness from underwater swimming 242
    unconsciousness from lack of oxygen 244

21 **gunshot and missile wounds 247**

    human missile wounds 247
    missile wounds of the blood vessels 248
    penetrating wounds of the great arteries of the chest 250

1
some general principles

First aid should not be rendered in a haphazard manner, even though such efforts may save human lives. More lives will be saved when aid is given on a systematic and knowledgeable basis, more suffering can be alleviated, further injury can be prevented, and greater protection in a legal sense can be achieved for all.

If the person who gives help knows in advance the most critical conditions and handles them in order from most to least serious he has the opportunity to do the most good in any accident or emergency situation. Standard first aid training alerts and educates the student to such responsibilities.

Medical readings that give greater understanding of emergency conditions can be considered from the viewpoint of the individual victim and his first aid needs, or from the viewpoint of commonly occurring injury-producing situations, such as the motor vehicle accident. The following readings represent only a very few of the professional articles available in the medical literature on the foregoing subjects, but they should provide a beginning for deeper understandings of emergency situations.

the severely injured patient

Shires, G. Tom and Ronald C. Jones. "Initial Management of the Severely Injured Patient," Journal of the American Medical Association, 213: 1872-1878, (No. 11), September 14, 1970.

Two surgeons of the University of Texas Southwestern Medical School in Dallas observed that *it is very important to classify injuries swiftly and to have an organized plan of management* when a victim is severely injured.

The surgeons suggest *three categories of injuries according to their severity,* as follows: 1) those which are an immediate threat to life, such as a gunshot wound or an obstructed airway, in which establishment of breathing and control of bleeding is primary. (This type of patient may require surgery within 5 to 10 minutes after arriving at the hospital); 2) those injuries which do not constitute an immediate threat to survival, such as gunshot wounds, stab wounds, or blunt injury to the chest or abdomen in which the victim's vital signs (respiration, heart rate and blood pressure) are stable (surgery may not be needed for one to two hours); and 3) those injuries in which the damage is hidden, such as may occur in blunt injury to the abdomen (hours or even days may permit laboratory studies, x-rays and other studies).

The *first and most important emergency measure is to establish effective breathing.* Treatment of shock may be started while someone else works with the airway. *Internal hemorrhage* requires immediate surgery once the victim has reached the hospital. The *control of external bleeding* is best accomplished by direct finger compression of the bleeding wound or vessel. Tourniquets are of little value for the control of major arterial bleeding and may be injurious if collateral or venous circulation is impaired.

All gunshot wounds of the abdomen are explored by the surgeon even if penetration is not obvious. Shock waves from the force of the bullet may cause internal damage to the bowel, liver, spleen or other part of the abdominal cavity without penetration of the bullet.

In some injuries *breathing may be obstructed* by mucus, fragments of bone, broken teeth, or dentures. *If the victim does not breathe normally after the upper airway has been cleared, injury to the chest must be suspected.* In chest injuries where the victim arrives in the emergency room in shock without evidence of blood loss, acute compression of the heart (cardiac tamponade) must be suspected by the surgeon. The compression may be due to bleeding into the pericardial sac around the heart from a blunt or penetrating injury. Fluid in the lungs, blood in the chest, a ruptured bronchial tube or major artery are also injuries that must be searched for by the physician in chest injuries. Broken ribs and a chest in which the lungs are collapsed may occur in chest injuries also. Positive pressure ventilation can expand the lungs and restore adequate breathing if the surgeon makes the proper diagnosis.

Damage to the arteries must be suspected if there has been a penetrating injury to any part of the body in the region of a major blood vessel. Early recognition of an injury to an artery is essential if the mobility of an extremity is to be saved.

A *combination of a head injury and the unconscious state* calls for an immediate establishment of an open airway so that breathing will be maintained. Extreme care must be taken in moving an unconscious patient until possible injuries to the spine have been evaluated. Low blood pressure seldom comes from an internal (closed) head injury, but almost always from the loss of blood in chest or abdominal injury. The physician can diagnose the cause of blood loss with abdominal or chest taps with an appropriate needle. In blunt injuries the urine must be examined for possible presence of blood since the kidney or bladder may be damaged.

Fractures must always be immobilized. Conversion of a closed fracture to an open one may be prevented by the application of an appropriate leg or arm splint. The management of chest or abdominal bleeding takes precedence over that of a fracture, unless along with the latter there is severe injury to an accompanying artery that may threaten the loss of life or limb.

multiple injuries from accidents

Wood, MacDonald, "Recognition of Multiple Injuries," Arizona Medicine, 25: 133-139 (No. 2), February 1968.

The Chairman of the Department of Surgery at the Maricopa County General Hospital in Phoenix, Arizona, says that the *primary needs for improvement in the care of injured persons are:* 1) the proper extrication of the victim from the accident; 2) the initial first aid treatment and 3) safe transportation of the injured person.

some general principles

It is tragic and illogical thinking to assume that if an accident victim is found with a broken bone, a bump on the head, or some other injury that the answer has been found to his entire problem. *The injured person is an emergency problem and he should always be considered as a multiple injury victim until it is proven otherwise.* A study at Cornell University has shown that 65 per cent of the persons in an automobile accident sustained injuries to two or more parts of the body. Another study of pedestrian accident victims showed that 80 per cent of 200 persons who were killed had suffered significant injury to two or more body areas. Fifty per cent of all those who had sustained abdominal injuries also had head injuries.

A rapid, careful and complete physical examination of an accident victim should determine the: 1) state of respiration; 2) extent of wounds; 3) extent of external bleeding; 4) presence of shock; 5) level of consciousness; 6) pupil response; 7) movements of the muscles of the face; 8) stability of the arms and legs, and 9) abdominal or pelvic tenderness. Spinal cord or vertebral injuries can be detected by testing the strength, motion and sensation of the extremities. Transient numbness or paralysis should alert the examiner to possible spinal cord injury and vertebral fracture or dislocation.

People with multiple injuries present a difficult problem and *those problems that offer the greatest threat to life should be treated first.* In evaluation of the injured a preferred order of priority would be to: 1) establish an *open airway* so that breathing can be assured; 2) control *bleeding;* 3) combat *shock;* 4) determine the extent of *chest injuries,* and 5) evaluate the *unconscious* patient.

An accurate history or description of the accident combined with repeated physical examination of the victim are needed in order to detect the injuries. It needs emphasis that every victim should be considered as having multiple injuries until proven otherwise, and that he is a *continuing diagnostic problem.* Laboratory and x-ray studies, as needed, should be done by the physician as an aid to diagnosis.

first aid for traffic victims

Pacy, Hanns. *"First Aid for Motorists,"* Medical Journal of Australia, 2-57th year: 280-283, (No. 6), August 8, 1970.

A physician of the Tea Gardens Memorial Hospital and Ambulance Trust of New South Wales believes that training in first aid should be a requirement for a driving license, because *a motorist is usually the first person to stop at the scene of a road accident* and because he must act rather than wait.

Dr. Pacy advocates *seven procedures if lives are to be saved, delays avoided, recovery assisted and later disabilities minimized.* The seven things that should be done are to: 1) note the time and place of the accident; 2) park one's own car correctly; 3) assess the situation quickly; 4) save lives if possible; 5) get whatever help is needed; 6) remove hazards or dangers; and 7) remove the victims from danger.

The *time and place of an accident should be noted and recorded* because witnesses may vary in their recollections, and excitement may obscure the memory of events.

The *motorist who sees an accident* should slow down gently, because the driver behind may not be aware of the situation. Parking room should be left for an ambulance, a tow truck, fire truck or other essential vehicles. The ignition key on your own car should be turned on to keep the right hand warning or turning light flickering. Cars on both sides of the highway should be parked to give warning in both directions.

In *assessing the accident situation* swiftly it should be determined if anyone is injured, unconscious, bleeding, or not breathing. Serious injuries should be distinguished from slight ones. It should also be decided if an ambulance or doctor is needed, if a rescue vehicle is needed for trapped victims and if all people in the accident have been accounted for.

Mouth-to-mouth *resuscitation, cardiac massage,* and application of a pad of cloth to *stop bleeding* should be done immediately if such procedures are needed.

Any unconscious person who is still breathing should be rolled on his side to stop the inhalation of blood or vomitus [unless spinal or other injuries make this procedure threatening.—Ed.].

Any *message sent for help* should be written down carefully for the messenger. Dr. Pacy recommends that every automobile should carry emergency message forms in triplicate. Inquiry should be made of stopped cars if they possess a two-way radio or trained personnel.

If the engine of the crashed car is still running it should be switched off, and smoking by bystanders should be discontinued. Traffic guards should be placed about 150 yards away in each direction to warn oncoming traffic. Flares and other warning signals should be used. No bystanders should be permitted to stand in such a way as to obscure lights of a parked car.

Injured persons in or out of damaged vehicles should be left to skilled personnel for removal unless there is danger from leaking gasoline or the victim is in a spot where he might be run over. Mouth-to-mouth resuscitation can be given to a person sitting in a car if necessary. *If an unconscious person has* collapsed in the seat of a car and his head has fallen forward so his breathing is obstructed, the airway must be freed by removal of dentures, blood, mucus or other materials while care is taken to protect the rescuer's fingers. The head may need to be moved gently to establish free breathing, with one hand under the chin and the other at the back of the head as the chin is eased forward until snoring or gargling stops. Someone must stay with such a victim until skilled help arrives.

Dr. Pacy believes *the most significant error almost invariably found at the scene of an accident* involves the unconscious person who has been left lying on his back where he may inhale blood, vomitus, or other materials, with a fatal outcome. [Spinal or other injuries may make movement of the patient hazardous.—Ed.]

In general, *immediate first aid should be restricted to the most urgently needed measures.*

immediate handling of traffic injuries

Kay, J. Albert and Lee T. Ford, "The Immediate Handling of Traffic Injuries," Missouri Medicine, 53: 285-87 (No. 4), April 1956.

J. Albert Key, M.D., and Lee T. Ford, M.D., from the Department of Surgery of the Washington University School of Medicine in St. Louis, Missouri, report on the difficulty of doing no further harm in the *handling of persons injured in traffic accidents.*

The victim should be removed from the vehicle if he cannot escape unaided. If he has an open wound and is bleeding copiously, *hemmorhage should be arrested as soon as possible.* In most instances, and especially in head and face wounds, this is best done by a pressure dressing. In this antibiotic age sterility of the emergency dressing is not as important as in the past because the patient is going to receive antibiotics and the wound will be cleansed and treated surgically within a few hours. Bacteria from the dressing will not have much chance to invade the tissues.

If the bleeding is from an extremity and the pressure dressing does not control it, a tourniquet should be improvised and applied. If the tourniquet is loosened at a subsequent time digital pressure should be applied over the severed vessel. A tourniquet should be used only when the bleeding cannot be controlled by a pressure dressing because the latter permits collateral circulation and this may save an extremity which might be lost if a tourniquet had been used for too long a time.

If the patient is unconscious, he should be lifted to the side of the road, turned on his side with the mouth down to facilitate drainage, and, if indicated, protected from the weather until an ambulance can take him to a hospital.

If the patient is lifted and carried to the side of the road *he should receive support to the middle of the spine as well as at both ends* and the body should be bent or stretched as little as possible. At least three persons should be used to lift the patient when this is necessary.

Major fractures should, if possible, be splinted before the patient is transported. This applies to both simple and compound fractures of the arm, forearm, hip, thigh, leg, and ankle. Transportation of patients with major fractures of long bones without splinting is not only painful to the patient, but increases the hemorrhage and shock and may cause increased damage to the soft tissues.

At the scene of the accident any person rendering first aid should: 1) see if the patient is living; 2) see that he has an open airway; 3) arrest serious hemorrhage; 4) arrange the patient comfortably; 5) cover any wound; 6) splint any major fractures of the extremities; 7) protect the patient from weather if this is necessary; and 8) handle the patient gently in order to avoid further injury during transportation.

Once the patient has been taken in the ambulance to the hospital he is in the hands of the surgeon who then assumes the responsibility for his proper treatment.

removal of persons injured in auto accidents

Kossuth, Louis C. "The Extrication of Victims from the Accident," Arizona Medicine, 26: 128-130, (No. 2), February 1969.

The Command Surgeon of the North American Air Defense Command says that *survival from a high speed collision may be directly related to the way in which an injured person is removed from his car.*

When an injured person is pinned, trapped, in an awkward unnatural position or not readily accessible in a small enclosed area inside a car, the *objective of extrication should be the initial movement of the victim in such a manner that an additional injury is not caused* or added to those injuries that the person may have sustained already.

The proper removal of a person injured in an automobile accident should involve a consideration of *the victim, the vehicle,* and *the environment.*

The vehicle accident accompanied by fire requires an immediate rescue. The technique of "grab and pull" must be accepted. On a high-speed highway the imminent hazard of a second collision may also justify the "grab and pull" approach, but there may be time for more careful consideration. If a vehicle is submerged beneath water, or is sinking, the "grab and pull" technique is necessary. If a vehicle is teetering on the brink of a cliff the same technique of rescue may be justified, but *the great majority of accidents occur with an environment that permits a calm, deliberate, planned removal of the victim from his car.*

Two factors are of significance: 1) the *injuries* that the victim has sustained, and 2) the *position* of the injured person. *Rapid examination* of the victim should be directed toward *two life-threatening injuries: respiratory difficulty and severe hemorrhage.* Respiratory difficulty demands first attention, but hemorrhage must be controlled to prevent shock. *After injuries to the victim have been assessed and treated, then the position of the injured person and the restrictive, restraining, or confining aspects* of the *collapse of the vehicle around the victim* can be determined. After the foregoing actions and assessments of the situation have been made the next question is: "How can this victim be moved with maximum gentleness and minimum risk of adding to his injuries?"

Three basic principles should be followed: 1) *rest is a basic factor* in the immediate treatment of many types of injuries; 2) *the car should be disentangled from the victim* and not the victim from the car; 3) it is always preferable to *put equipment on the patient rather than move the victim onto the equipment.* A person with a back injury in a bucket seat should be removed from his car by releasing the seat and removing it with the victim still seated until he reaches the hospital. Damage to nerves, blood vessels, later non-union of broken bones and infections may occur when victims with broken bones are moved without first being splinted. *Splints should be applied in the car before removal of the victim.* The Thomas splint is best, but rolled magazines or a board can do the job. Ambulance drivers in particular need special training for victim removal.

transportation of accident victims

Webb, Roscoe C. "Transportation of Accident Victims," Modern Medicine, 20: 68-70, (No. 17), September 1, 1952.

Roscoe C. Webb, M.D., of the University of Minnesota, reports that the Committee on Trauma of the American College of Surgeons has annually been investigating first aid and transportation of the injured in five cities. Thus far, *the Committee has found conditions shockingly chaotic.*

Injuries resulting from fractures are not limited to those occurring at the time of the accident. Unwise attempts to use the injured extremity may cause or increase displacement of fragments, increase the injuries to soft parts, and perhaps lead to penetration of the skin by the ends of the bone. Large blood vessels may be torn and exposed ends of bones may become contaminated with dirt and other particles. Frequently there is jolting and other damage during the time the accident victim is being transferred to the hospital or doctor's office. He may even receive insufficient protection as he is lifted to and from the x-ray table and as he is being given an anesthetic.

The proper procedure is in direct contrast to this. *The man with a broken leg should remain where he is until a proper splint can be applied,* or at least until he can have someone pull hard on his foot as he is being lifted and carried, and should be examined thoroughly but gently.

Several cities have adopted ordinances for regulation of ambulance services. Typically the ordinance specifies minimum equipment to be carried and minimum training of personnel in first aid and application of splints, and sets forth penalties for noncompliance.

For passage of an ambulance ordinance, it is first advisable to obtain the official support of the local medical society.

The next step is to educate those who operate the ambulances, both public and private. When ambulance attendants find that the medical profession is interested in helping them with the practical applications of modern methods for the transportation of injured patients, they generally adopt the plan without objection.

After the ambulance organizations have become equipped with transportation splints and the attendants have learned how to apply them, other improved methods naturally follow. Some ambulances, for example, may carry oxygen and blood plasma as further refinements.

wound healing

Ehrlich, H. Paul and Thomas K. Hunt. "Effects of Cortisone and Vitamin A on Wound Healing," Annals of Surgery, 167: 324-328 (No. 3), March 1968.

Two members of the Department of Surgery of the University of California School of Medicine report *a study on the process of wound healing.*

In a wound, *inflammation and the inflammatory phase are somehow essential to the healing process.* Thus, inflammatory cells, ground substance, fibroblasts (connective tissue cells that support and bind tissues of all sorts), collagen (a supportive protein), regenerating capillaries (small blood vessels that repair or renew themselves), and epithelial migration (movement of internal and external coverings of body parts, such as the skin and internal linings of vessels and other parts) are all involved in the process of healing of a wound.

When *cortisone* is given in moderate or large amounts within the first two or three days after injury it delays the appearance of almost all the elements that are needed for healing. Like cortisone, other anti-inflammatory steroids also delay the healing process. These steroids do not delay healing if they are given after the third day from the injury.

A lysosome is one of the very small bodies that can be seen under the electron microscope in many types of cells. *The lysosome contains various enzymes which are released when there is injury to the cell. These enzymes take a prominent part in the inflammatory process, and thus are involved in the first steps of wound healing.*

It is possible that cortisone (and other steroids) increase the integrity of the lysosome, so that the enzymes contained therein are not released as they would normally be following injury. Thus, the action of cortisone on the prevention or alleviation of inflammation may reflect its action on lysosomes.

Vitamin A, on the other hand, has been found to make the lysosome more unstable; thus it could be reasoned that Vitamin A might counteract the theoretical action of cortisone on lysosome and might thereby permit normal healing of a wound, even though cortisone is present.

The two surgeons in this investigation used cortisone to delay wound healing in experimental animals, then added Vitamin A and found that healing returned to normal. However, when Vitamin A was used alone it did not increase wound healing. Thus, the action of Vitamin A on wound healing appeared to lie in its prevention of the effects of cortisone. The study does appear to support the importance of lysosome in healing.

Despite much research, the details of the metabolism of healing wounds are not completely known. The wounded tissues themselves may supply vital nutritional elements needed for healing. Some substances are rapidly synthesized in the healing wound. Deficiencies of various kinds can be expected to impair the process of wound healing.

application of cold to injuries

Vernon, Sidney. "Injury, Ice and Compression," Connecticut State Medical Journal, 21: 111-12 (No. 2), February 1957.

Sidney Vernon, M.D., of Willimantic, Connecticut, observes that the *use of cold in the treatment of injury may be unique* in inhibiting simultaneously pain, exudation, thrombosis, shock, infection, toxic absorption, and tissue devitalization.

The standard use of cold combined with compresssion may be advantageous in special conditions. A compressive dressing which controls bleeding may be lifesaving, yet pressure on anemic or devitalized tissue is not safe. Devitalized tissue may incubate bacteria and warmth would accelerate this process. The use of cold to inhibit bacterial growth in devitalized tissue is more ideal.

Shock may occur after the release of a tourniquet; *use of cold may minimize this ill effect.*

Ice applied to an ankle fracture even for a short period slows the swelling and a compression dressing helps to control interstitial oozing. With ice and compression, there is less chance that the time taken before manipulation or x-ray will jeopardize the quality of the result.

2
cardiac emergencies

The speed and manner in which the heart attack victim is brought to first aid and medical care can make the difference between life and death. Mobile units for the heart attack victim may or may not be needed in a particular community, but the fundamental principle of immediate professional care persists in any locality.

There are various kinds of heart attacks and multiple causes of heart disturbances. There is a great range in severity from the least to the most significant. The layman, or even many first aiders, might reach the conclusion that death has ensued when the heart stops, but such is not necessarily the case. In some cases the heart can be induced to beat again to preserve life and vitality for the victim.

mobile units for heart attack victims

Pyo, Yoon H. and Richard W. Watts. "A Mobile Coronary Care Unit: An Evaluation for Its Need," Annals of Internal Medicine, 73: 61-66, (No. 1), July 1970.

Two physicians of the Coronary Care Unit, Fairview General Hospital in Cleveland, Ohio, observe that *intensive medical attention for heart patients in hospitals has reduced the death rate by about one-half* in persons suffering from myocardial infarction (bleeding into the heart muscle from a broken blood vessel or damage to the heart muscle from a blod clot) *in the coronary care units* of the hospital.

However, the two physicians report, *these coronary care units can do nothing* for approximately 250,000 Americans who will die from heart attacks per year before they arrive at the emergency room of a hospital. Sixty per cent of the deaths from this form of heart disease (myocardial infarction) occur within one hour of the attack.

Since 1966 mobile intensive care units for heart patients have been in operation in some cities, and others are being planned.

This report by Doctors Pyo and Watts *covers a study of 87 patients as to whether or not the cost of a mobile coronary unit is worth the great cost in money and skilled personnel in terms of the results obtained.*

For the majority of heart attack patients the *delay in securing intensive medical care comes from the failure of the patient to seek prompt medical help* rather than a lack of immediate transportation to a hospital. The first reaction of many patients to a critical chest pain is to deny that it is serious, probably to defend family members from anxiety. This delay in seeking help is the primary cause of not getting proper care, and *it is this delay than can be shortened only by education,* rather than by the availability of a mobile heart unit. *Each community should decide for itself* whether or not a mobile coronary unit is needed. It may be that better training of rescue squads and ambulance personnel can make the expensive mobile coronary unit unnecessary. *In West Cleveland there are seven rescue squads that can reach 90 per cent of the patients within 15 minutes after receiving a call.* If only one centrally located mobile coronary care unit is available it may take a greater time to reach the patient. *Education of the victim or his family to call for help immediately is most important* especially in those cases where mobile coronary care units are not available.

first aid for heart attacks

Kelly, James H. "Cardiac Emergencies," *Journal-Lancet,* 85: 181-185, (No. 5), May 1965.

An attending physician of the Veterans Hospital at St. Cloud, Minnesota observes that although more deaths occur from heart disease in this country than from any other cause, *many lives could be saved* in some heart attacks if the proper emergency care were given.

Obviously, *the greatest need of a patient suffering from a heart attack is for medical care,* but the kind of heart attack that is involved has much to do with the chances of recovery.

In the blocking of a blood vessel to the heart itself (coronary occlusion) with subsequent death of a part of the heart muscle because of a lack of oxygen and nutrients (myocardial infarction), there is typically a crushing or pressure pain under the sternum and radiating to one or both arms, neck, jaw, or back. Pain in the left area of the chest above the breast is most common. Often the pain is accompanied by sweating and difficult breathing. The pain may last from a few minutes to several hours. *Relief of pain and anxiety, an adequate supply of oxygen, and treatment for shock are the greatest needs of the person* suffering from this kind of a heart attack. Relief from pain is the most immediate need, and *morphine* injected by a physician probably gives the best relief. Relief of pain helps to control shock from the heart attack. *Oxygen* is best supplied by a mask over the face or tubes in the nose. This kind of emergency treatment can be obtained only in the hospital or the doctor's office. In this type of heart attack the best first aid is a swift call of a physician.

Disturbances of heart rhythm are very common. A normal heart can withstand increases in the heart rate up to 180 beats per minute for 24 to 48 hours without serious consequences, but an experience of this kind can be a great source of anxiety for the victim. It is usual for such sudden increases in the heart rate to stop just as suddenly as they begin. An increase in heart rate commonly occurs in young people who have no heart disease. *Prolonged holding of the breath* may stop such an attack. If not, *induced vomiting*, such as putting a finger down the throat, may succeed in stopping the accelerated heart rate. *Massage of the principal artery of the neck* (involving the carotid sinus) may help stop the attack. Accelerated heart rates that do not respond to such simple first aid procedures should be quickly referred to a physician.

When the heart stops (ventricular standstill), external cardiac massage may induce the heart to beat again. Mouth-to-mouth artificial respiration is also very important for supplying adequate oxygen to the person with this kind of heart attack.

In all cases of heart attack the best first aid procedure is to call a physician at once.

external cardiac compression

Thaler, Manning Michael. "External Cardiac Compression," Pediatrics, 31: 303-310, (No. 2), February 1963.

A physician at the the Hospital for Sick Children in Toronto, Canada observes that the emergency maneuver known as closed-chest cardiac massage or external cardiac compression has been widely accepted by both medical and lay personnel since 1960 in the treatment of cardiac standstill.

Dr. Thaler observes that *this technique may also be used in conditions of shock* where the maintenance of a strong pulse is of prime importance.

It is difficult to define cardiac arrest precisely, but Dr. Thaler believes that any (pediatric) patient without a pulse or precordial heartbeat should be immediately treated with external cardiac compression.

The only contraindications are pneumothorax (air or gas in the pleural cavity resulting in *lung collapse)* and intrathoracic hemorrhage *(bleeding inside the chest).* An interval of even 4 minutes may result in irreversible damage to the central nervous system. *Of equal importance is maintenance of ventilation* by mouth-to-mouth breathing or appropriate other technique (face mask or intubation).

The following technique for cardiac compression is recommended by Dr. Thaler:

(1) *The patient should be lying on a hard surface on his back* with the head about 10 degrees below the horizontal plane.

(2) *The heel of one hand is placed on the lower sternum but not on the ziphoid cartilage.* Infants may be resuscitated by two fingers only, and young children with one hand only, but the other hand may be used atop the first if needed.

(3) The sternum is depressed vertically about 3 to 5 centimeters downward with a moderate thrust or push. Gradual squeezing is not effective.

(4) Compression is repeated about 50 times per minute. The lungs should be inflated about every 4 compressions at this pace.

(5) Treatment should be continued for about one hour. Dilation of the pupils indicates an insufficient blood supply to the brain. The pulse (femoral or carotid) should also be checked.

(6) If possible an E.K.G. should be taken.

About 3,000 to 10,000 cases of cardiac arrest occur in the United States each year. About one adult in 1500 to 2500 who have surgical operations under general anesthesia suffers cardiac arrest. The rate may be higher in infants.

Complications such as broken ribs, hemorrhage of the liver, fractured sternum, injury to the heart or major blood vessels may occur with hemorrhage into the chest and other complications (such as bone marrow emboli) may occur, but the possibility of saving a "dead" person outweighs the risk of injury. *Proper instruction cuts down on complications.* Only moderate force should be applied to the chest. In newborn infants blood pressures of 70 mm. Hg. have been produced by compression with the tips of two fingers. Excessive pressures and pressures over the wrong areas of the chest appear to be responsible for most injuries.

[IMPORTANT NOTE: *Because of the serious nature of the complications that may occur from the improper application of external cardiac massage, it is recommended that the technique should not be taught to elementary school children or to junior high school pupils. Only mature senior high school students and college students or adults can probably be trusted with a careful application of external cardiac massage. Fortunately, the occasion for its use should seldom occur, so the hazard of improper application should not arise too frequently.—Ed.*]

external cardiac massage

Baringer, J. Richard, Edwin W. Salzman, Wallace A. Jones and Allan L. Friedlich. *"External Cardiac Massage,"* **New England Journal of Medicine, 265: 62-65, (No. 2), July 13, 1961.**

Four physicians of the Harvard Medical School and the Massachusetts General Hospital in Boston report on their experience with *84 patients on whom external cardiac massage was used* in an effort to revive the heart beat and circulation of the blood.

External cardiac massage is a simple process which requires no special equipment, but because *complications from its use can occur* it should be used only on unconscious persons in whom the heart has stopped (thus stopping the circulation of the blood). The patient should be lying on his back, preferably on a hard surface. One hand of the person attempting to revive the victim should be placed across the chest immediately over the lower sternum. The other hand should be placed atop the first so that pressure can be brought to bear on the lower part of the sternum. This pressure should be exerted at a rate of 60 to 90 times per minute with a force sufficient to cause the sternum to move toward the back or vertebral column a distance of about 1 to 1½ inches each compression. This rapid, up and down compression should be applied only over the sternum in order to avoid soft-tissue injury and breaking of the ribs. The resuscitator can watch the effectiveness of his revival efforts by closely observing the femoral pulse and the size of the pupils. Good results are being achieved when the pupils do not dilate and the femoral pulse is reestablished.

In this series of 84 persons in whom the heart had stopped, good pulses or undilated pupils (or both) were obtained in 38 cases; in 36 cases an effective, spontaneous heartbeat was resumed; in 10 cases fibrillation of the heart was stopped; in 15 cases recovery of consciousness was achieved; in 23 cases the patient survived for over 3 hours, and in 4 cases the patients survived to leave the hospital. The patients who did not survive were suffering from serious and severe disorders that subsequently caused their deaths.

Complications from external cardiac massage included the breaking of ribs, hemorrhage into the lung cavity, bleeding into the covering of the heart itself; serious injury to the liver and the blocking of blood vessels by bone marrow. (Obviously *this method of revival of heart and circulation should be used only in extreme emergencies* in which the heart has already stopped and death is a foregone conclusion if something is not done to revive the heart and circulation.) Pressure on the lower part of the sternum only and not on the nearby ribs or other tissues seems to be the best method for prevention of injuries from use of external cardiac massage.

broken ribs from external cardiac massage

Henriksen, Hans. "Rib Fractures Following External Cardiac Massage," Acta Anaesthesiologica, 11: 57-64 (Fasc. 1), 1967.

A staff member of the Copenhagen County Hospital In Denmark reports on an investigation of rib fractures caused by external cardiac massage in 37 patients who came to the autopsy table after death.

In a first report on the use of external cardiac massage in 1960 no mention was made that rib fractures might be a hazard in attempting to revive persons whose hearts had stopped. However, since that date *numerous investigators have described hazards from broken ribs in the use of this life-saving procedure.*

In this particular study, external cardiac massage had been performed by various medical personnel, including ambulance drivers, physicians, and anaesthetists. *The duration of the emergency procedure was from 25 seconds to 175 minutes on different patients.*

In 97 percent of the patients who were 20 years of age or older, rib fractures were found by post mortem examination to have occurred. Of 8 persons *under the age of 20 years no rib fractures were found,* but at all other ages (one victim was over 80) fractures of the ribs were found. *The older the victim the greater the average number of broken ribs.* The 80-year old person, for example, had 19 broken ribs and those between the ages of 70 to 80 years had an average of 9 broken ribs per person. Persons between the ages of 20 to 30 years, however, had only 2 broken ribs per person. *Fracture of the sternum itself was present in 24 percent of the cases.*

It has been determined that the sternum must be pressed inwards about 4 to 5 centimeters (about 1.5 inches or more) to achieve compression of the heart sufficient to achieve an adequate movement of blood from the heart. *Experiments have shown that ribs may be broken with as little compression of the sternum as 2 centimeters.*

It has been shown from this study that *a fracture of the rib may occur with the very first compressions.* When the ribs are broken closer to the side of the chest wall (rather than at their attachment to the sternum) the broken, jagged edges represent a greater hazard to the life and health of the victim. In one instance the liver had been perforated by the sharp edge of a broken rib. Other hemorrhages into the chest had occurred from rib injuries.

The investigators concluded that *any patient whose heart has stopped, and who receives external cardiac massage, must be considered as a chest-injury case if he survives.* Even if the chest injury is a mild one, treatment must be directed against the almost inevitable injury.

cessation of breathing and heart action

Editorial. *"Resuscitation," British Medical Journal, 279-80, (No. 5326), February 2, 1963.*

British medical authorities state that *within 3 to 5 minutes at normal body temperature irreversible changes have occurred in the brain with cessation of heart action and respiration.* After 10 minutes reanimation is improbable. Clinical death occurs with stoppage of both heart and respiration. Biological death occurs about 10 minutes later.

The interval between clinical death and biological death may be prolonged by four methods:

(1) Cardiac massage with *artificial respiration.*

(2) Hypothermia *(lowering of body temperature)*.

(3) Circulation of the blood by a pump oxygenator outside the body.

(4) Hyperbaric *oxygen in a pressure chamber.*

External cardiac massage combined with mouth-to-mouth breathing may maintain circulation to the brain while the patient is being taken to the hospital.

Lowering the body temperature delays glycolysis (the hydrolysis of sugar in the body) in the brain. When the body temperature is lowered to 77 degrees F. (as compared to the normal 98.6 degrees) the energy potential of the brain after 30 minutes of cardiac arrest is equal to that of 5 to 6 minutes at normal temperature. At 60 minutes all energy potential has been exhausted. The Russians have supported life in dogs for two hours with cardiac arrest and with subsequent recovery by reducing body temperature to 50 to 54 degrees F.

Oxygen has been supplied under pressure of two to three atmospheres in the management of terminal conditions.

Recovery from an inanimate state has been achieved after 45 minutes when the body temperature has been lowered to about 50 degrees F. but circulation of the blood outside the body has been maintained.

sudden deaths of athletes

James, Thomas N., Peter Froggatt and Thomas K. Marshall. "Sudden Death in Young Athletes," Annals of Internal Medicine, 67: 1013-1021, (No. 5), November 1967.

Three physicians from the Section on Cardiovascular Research of the Henry Ford Hospital in Detroit, Michigan report that although *sudden unexpected death of a young athlete is not an unfamiliar event,* there are often few medical facts to report by the attending physician.

In such deaths there are limited possible mechanisms that may be responsible for the fatality. A *sudden disturbance of the heart rhythm is one of these mechanisms.* For this reason the three physicians recently studied the hearts of two young athletes who died suddenly although previously considered to be in good health and in whom autopsy provided no explanation of the death. In both cases, detailed studies of the hearts showed that only these organs were abnormal, and in both cases the conduction system of the heart was at fault (in other words, the rhythm of the heart would be disturbed).

In one case an 18-year old football player felt well before a game and cycled eight miles with his brother to the game. After 10 minutes of participation in the game he said to his brother, who was also playing, that he felt very tired. About 30 seconds later he collapsed and within a few minutes, on admission to a local hospital that was located beside the football field, he was dead. On special study after death, only the heart was found to be abnormal and it was the conduction system of the heart (which controls heart rhythm) that was impaired.

In the other case a 15-year old boy was playing with five companions on some grassy waste land in team wrestling matches. After 10 or 15 minutes of play the boy sat down and said that he felt sick. He lay on his back and turned blue. Two men were called, one of whom tried artificial respiration while the other called an ambulance. The boy was unconscious but still alive when the ambulance arrived, but he was dead on arrival at the hospital. Special study of the heart revealed that it was normal except for the conduction system.

According to these three physicians, the most important practical point of the foregoing observations is the probability that under ideal conditions both boys could have been saved. *Appropriate treatment could have produced complete recovery.*

Conditions during athletic games are not always ideal, particularly in rural and other isolated areas, but a number of sudden deaths of young athletes have occurred within a short distance of medical facilities. Some physicians with a special interest in sports medicine may have considered *the possibility of a disturbance of cardiac rhythm as a cause of sudden death,* but it is probably accurate to say that many have not. The possibility *should be considered always,* in addition to more obvious cardiac injuries, whenever a young athlete collapses suddenly. In both of the cases reported above the general condition of the heart was good and with normal electrical activity life and vigor should have been sustained.

causes of disturbances in rhythm of the heart

Harkavy, Joseph. "Cardiac Arrhythmias due to Hypersensitivity: A Report of Ten Cases," Journal of the Mount Sinai Hospital, 36: 485-496, (No. 6), Nov.-Dec. 1969.

An Emeritus Clinical Professor of Medicine of the Mount Sinai School of Medicine in New York City reports on his experience with ten patients who had *heart disorders caused by stimulation by and allergic sensitivity to certain foods, pollens, coffee, alcohol and tobacco.*

Most of the patients experienced heart attacks (irregularities of rhythm) after eating certain foods, drinking alcohol or coffee, or smoking tobacco.

Nine of the 10 patients in this study had no evidence of heart disease. All, however, had heart attacks of irregularities in rhythm after exposure to certain substances to which they appeared to be unduly sensitive.

Beneath the reactions was a solid association with allergy. The allergic origin of the disturbances of heart rhythm was established, to the satisfaction of Dr. Harkavy, by: 1) a personal or family history of allergy; 2) respiratory or other evidence of allergy; 3) positive skin reactions to certain allergy tests; 4) verification of heart attacks after exposure to substances, to which the patient was allergic, by means of repeated clinical tests, and 5) complete cessation and control of the heart disturbances by removal of the offending food or pollen to which the patient had been found to be allergic.

Fibrillation (irregular contractions of the heart muscle), if uncontrolled, overworks the heart and may cause enlargment or other complication in a heart that is otherwise free from disease. Finding of disturbances of heart rhythm in people with normal hearts who have hay fever or asthma suggests that allergy may have a relationship to the problem.

In this study, nine of the 10 patients had no heart disease, but did have extra beats, a fast pulse (tachycardia) that originated above the ventricles of the heart, and atrial fibrillation (an irregular rhythm of the muscles of the upper part of the heart).

In some allergic persons, according to Dr. Harkavy, *the only shock organ (point of special stress) may be the heart.* To diagnose this origin of heart disorders the physician needs to base his judgment on clinical symptoms, an allergic study, and an EKG (electrocardiogram).

In this report of 10 patients the *heart attacks were most evident during the grass pollen season and after the eating of milk, chocolate, apples or cheese.* When these foods were eliminated from the diet or the patient was desensitized to pollens, the attacks disappeared, as confirmed by EKG studies. Some specific examples follow.

case histories

1 A 32-year-old woman had irregularities of heart rhythm for nine years; they were precipitated by either alcohol or tobacco. Control was achieved by elimination of these substances.

2 A 10-year old child with hives and other disorders of the skin due to allergy had severe attacks of rapid beating of the heart (rates of 160 to 180 per minute) during pollen seasons, but had recoveries during other seasons. He also had attacks of heart irregularities when chocolate or oranges were consumed. After these foods were eliminated from the diet he was free from attacks of tachycardia for four years.

3 A 5-year old child had attacks of a fast heart rate and hives whenever he ate chocolate. Without chocolate he had no heart irregularities.

4 A 33-year old patient had severe tachycardia whenever he smoked tobacco or drank alcohol during a period of 11 years. An immediate severe reaction would come from the drinking of two cups of coffee; this was confirmed with EKG studies. Use of an antihistamine (Benadryl), which is helpful in the treatment of allergy, would terminate the attacks within 10 minutes.

5 A 48-year old patient had a marked food sensitivity, although he had had no hay fever. He would develop severe atrial fibrillation after smoking, or after eating certain foods, especially shellfish or spices. The heart irregularities disappeared after these foods were eliminated from his diet. Later the patient had heart attacks from tree pollens; these were eliminated for five years after desensitization to grasses, tree pollens, and dust as well as the offending foods.

The basic conclusion of Dr. Harkavy was that heart symptoms due to antigen-antibody reactions in the heart muscles, involving the release of histamine, may cause heart disorders. Since antihistamines usually controlled these heart attacks, he believes that any person with irregularities in the beating of the heart should be investigated from the standpoint of allergies.

3
cessation of breathing

When breathing has ceased, the first aider has less than 10 minutes in which to save the life of a human without permanent damage to the brain from lack of oxygen. The application of mouth-to-mouth breathing is the most efficient procedure the first aider can use in most emergency situations of this nature, but it is not the only form of artificial respiration. Circumstances may dictate the use of another.

Whatever method is used for the restoration of breathing, it must be emphasized that so long as artificial respiration is being provided for the victim that he *is breathing,* although not by his own volition, and that damage may be prevented and a life may be saved so long as breathing of any kind continues.

fundamental mechanisms in breathing

Editorial. "Control of Breathing," British Medical Journal, 3: 720-721, (No. 5725), September 26, 1970.

A medical member of the staff of the British Medical Journal discusses *the complicated process by which a human responds to a lack of oxygen.* A simplified version follows.

Whenever there is a deficiency of oxygen, breathing is immediately stimulated. *The acceleration of breathing occurs because cells that are sensitive to changes in the oxygen and carbon dioxide levels of the blood inform parts of the brain of these changes.* These cells are known as *chemoreceptors* and obviously they must be located in the circulatory system, where they are known as the aortic and carotid chemoreceptors.

The carotid body is composed of islands of tissue separated by wide channels through which blood flows. The carotid body has a system of nerves that carries messages to the brain and which control its own blood flow and oxygen consumption. The *chemoreceptors respond* not only to a fall in *blood oxygen,* but also to a rise in blood carbon dioxide and to a change in the *acidity of the blood* (hydrogen ion activity). As a consequence, whenever a person suffers from a deficiency of oxygen his *central nervous system* (brain) begins a drive toward better ventilation (breathing).

When a person is born at high altitudes this ventilatory drive is blunted and no correction is achieved even though the person may live for many years at sea level. Conversely, a person who is born at sea level and moves to high altitudes maintains this acute drive to increased ventilation whenever there is a lack of oxygen.

A slow ventilatory acclimatization occurs over several days when the lack of oxygen (such as at high altitude) persists. This adjustment appears to depend on an ability of the brain to conduct its metabolism under conditions of reduced oxygen.

When the chemoreceptors are damaged, an acute lack of oxygen depresses ventilation rather than accentuates it. The same effect is produced when the sympathetic nervous system is impaired by drugs or disease and severe falls in blood flow to the brain aggravate the lack of oxygen. A rise in the arterial carbon dioxide level acidifies *the cerebrospinal fluid* and stimulates a *chemoreceptor* in that fluid which in turn stimulates breathing.

Some people with severe bronchitis appear to have an impairment of their ventilatory drive, and deficiency of oxygen early in life may produce a permanent injury to this mechanism.

artificial respiration

Council on Physical Medicine. "Resuscitation," Journal of the American Medical Association, 138: 23-24, (No. 1), September 4, 1948.

A joint statement issued by the Council on Physical Medicine and the American National Red Cross in 1948 pointed out that there are many ways of giving artificial respiration. But *in asphyxia it is vitally important that artificial respiration be started without a moment's delay.* Most victims of asphyxia will die if delay occurs in providing resuscitation while apparatus is being brought to the scene or medical help is being obtained. Accordingly, the general public should be taught a method for giving artificial respiration that can be administered without apparatus of any kind.

The following are important points to bear in mind:

(1) A nonbreathing person should be given artificial respiration immediately by the most convenient method at hand.

(2) The air passages must be free from obstruction. The tongue sometimes presses back into the pharynx, shutting off the airway. The first aider should insert two fingers far back into the mouth and press downward and forward on the tongue. Thus the tongue is brought into proper position. Fluid or vomitus may also obstruct the passageway somewhat. It may be advisable to wipe out the mouth, reaching far back with a handkerchief.

These measures of bringing the tongue forward and of removing other obstructions should be accomplished at once.

(3) If a person has not been breathing for five or ten minutes, the chance of survival is slight, even if the most efficient inhalators or resuscitators are used. Nevertheless, an attempt at resuscitation should be made when the slightest chance for recovery exists. Artificial respiration should never be stopped when a pulse or heartbeat can be felt. Recovery of normal breathing may be long delayed, especially in cases of electric shock.

Most patients recover within about half an hour, but some have been resuscitated after several hours of artificial respiration.

survival with artificial respiration

Ross, Bernard D. "Five Year Survey of Methods for Artificial Respiration," Journal of the American Medical Association, 129:443-47, (No. 6), October 6, 1945.

Bernard D. Ross, M.D., Ph.D., of Miami, Florida, reports on a five-year survey of methods for artificial respiration.

Artificial respiration is a form of therapy which does not readily lend itself to clinical study. *Acute asphyxia requires immediate treatment if the patient is to recover,* and seconds may mean the difference between recovery and death. As a result, laymen cannot wait for the arrival of the physician before instituting treatment, and rarely does a physician arrive before the critical period of treatment is over.

Experimental work has been done in this field, but the results are not generally accepted as being conclusive.

There is good reason to doubt that values for the respiratory exchange in normal subjects have any bearing on the exchange in the deeply asphyxiated individual whose muscles are atonic and without resilience. This is especially true of the Schafer prone pressure method, which depends on elastic recoil of the diaphragm for production of inspiration. The method of Killick and Eve is unique in that it does not depend on elastic recoil. In this method the patient is alternately tipped back and forth on a stretcher, the weight of the viscera causing the diaphragm to move back and forth as a piston. This method is under trial in England but has not been used to any extent in this country. [Note date of this report.—Ed.]

For fourteen years the Council on Physical Medicine has been investigating methods, both manual and mechanical, recommended for the administration of artifical respiration.

Reports of cases of artificial respiration were collected from the United States Coast Guard and from the Chicago, Los Angeles, and Detroit fire departments during the years 1940 through 1944. These organizations sent in reports on all cases, regardless of whether or not resuscitation occurred. A total of 3,352 reports were obtained.

Among these were *153 cases of acute asphyxia in which a resuscitator, a mechanical device for artificial respiration employing alternate blowing and sucking, resulted in revival.* None of the patients, 80 of whom were newborn infants, showed evidences of injury as a result of this procedure.

In 58 cases of acute asphyxia in which the Schafer prone pressure method was used either entirely or in part there were no reports of fractured ribs. Such injuries have been said to be a possible result of improper use of this method.

No instance of revival was reported in which more than fifteen minutes elapsed between the cessation of breathing and the start of artificial respiration.

The survival rate was poorest for cases of electric shock, and best for asphyxia of the newborn. Ratios of survivals to deaths for various conditions in which artificial respiration was attempted are indicated in the following table.

Condition	Survivals	Deaths
Electric shock	0	16.0
Heart attacks	1	42.7
Suffocation	1	10.5
Drowning	1	2.7
Carbon monoxide poisoning	1	2.2
Asphyxia of the newborn	1	1.2

It is only in cases of immersion that there are enough data to permit any type of comparison. In 82 cases of immersion in which the Schafer method was used there were 35 survivals. In 44 cases of immersion in which a resuscitator was used there were only two survivals and in both of these cases the Schafer method was used prior to the use of resuscitator. It seems probable that much of this apparent superiority of the Schafer method in cases of immersion is due to the fact that no precious seconds were wasted in waiting for the arrival of a mechanical apparatus. *It cannot be emphasized too strongly that an asphyxiated person must have artificial respiration at once. Waiting for a machine, however efficient the machine may be, is apt to be fatal.*

the eve method of artificial respiration

Eve, Frank C. "Resuscitation of the Drowned Today," Journal of the American Medical Association, 124:964-67, (No. 14), April 1, 1944.

Frank C. Eve, M.D., of London, England, says that our implicit faith in Schafer's method of artificial respiration was shaken by Surgeon Commander Gibbens, who wrote that in the Royal Navy this method was rarely successful, although practiced by trained hands. [Note date of report.—Ed.]

This lack of response in bad drowning cases is due to lack of muscular tone, and this in turn is due to asphyxia of the nerve cells, which maintain tone and respiration. The main respirating agent is a thin sheet of muscle (the diaphragm) at the base of the lungs. In health this is pulled up into a dome by the elastic contraction of the lungs. When the diaphragm contracts its dome is lowered and air is pulled into the chest. But when the diaphragm loses its tone progressively, as in drowning, it is pulled up by the elastic lungs into a position of extreme expiration. Schafer's method would then be useless, especially as it depends entirely on the elastic tone (no longer present) of muscles for inspiration when the pressure of the hands is taken off the patient's back. Schafer naturally assumed in 1908 that his method, which works well in normal conscious persons, would also work in the almost drowned, but this unfortunately is not true.

In 1932 Dr. Eve was called to render medical service to a two-year-old girl, propped up in bed and dying with a death rattle (mucus surging to and fro in the windpipe). He noticed that the diaphragm was not working, and inquiry revealed that the girl had recovered from diphtheria six weeks previously and had been well until her breathing went wrong a few hours before.

In cases of "death rattle" Dr. Eve was in the habit of tilting his patients so that the windpipe sloped downhill in order that the mucus might drain into the throat from where it could be swabbed. This tilt cured the death rattle in a few minutes, but the physician reflected that it would compress the lungs and thus conduce to pneumonia if continuous. He asked if there were a rocking chair in the house so that the head-up and head-down posture could be alternated. A long rocking chair was available to which a platform of folded blankets was added and the child tied on.

The devoted parents alternated the tilt a dozen times a minute so the weight of the abdominal contents pulled and pushed the diaphragm up and down like a piston. This completely relieved the child's breathing until the diaphragm paralysis passed off after two and a half days. She is still alive and healthy. In this interesting way, Dr. Eve stumbled on a new method of resuscitation by rocking.

Faced by the failures of Schafer's method, the British Navy in 1943 turned to the rocking method, which worked by gravity and was independent of muscular tone. The method was adapted to ships by fixing, under the middle of an ordinary stretcher, a pair of grooved wooden blocks to prevent slipping. On these the stretcher could be rocked 45 degrees each way, either on a trestle 34 inches high or on a loop of rope slung from the hammock hooks. Schafer's method is used at first until rocking can actually begin. The patient is laid face downward and the ankles and wrists are lashed to the handles of the stretcher. The first head-down tilt of 45 degrees is maintained till no more water drains from stomach or lungs. After a few minutes a tilt of 30 degrees each way (ten times a minute) is enough to ventilate the lungs. The advantages are that untrained operators can work the rocker. It cannot injure ribs or viscera and is independent of muscular tone in blood vessels or diaphragm, in which respect Schafer's method fails. Wet clothes can be removed during rocking and warmth applied.

Blood falls from the lungs past the open valves of the left side of the heart into the arteries of the trunk and legs. Hence, in rocking, gravity propels the blood alternately in arteries and veins; reflux is prevented by valves in the veins and heart. Blood flow to the brain can be kept going by alternation of head-up and head-down positions.

Resuscitation of the drowned is not merely working the bellows of the lungs but a fight to revive cold asphyxiated nerve cells by a circulation of warm blood oxygenated by moving lungs.

inadequacy of the schafer method of artificial respiration

Comroe, Julius H., Jr., and Robert D. Dripps. *"Artificial Respiration," Journal of the American Medical Association, 130: 381-83, (No. 7), February 16, 1946.*

Julius H. Comroe, Jr., M.D., and Robert D. Dripps, M.D., of Philadelphia, report a study of the relative effectiveness of the Schafer and Eve methods of artificial respiration in the resuscitation of two patients.

In these two patients there was a complete respiratory arrest. In one patient respiration ceased following a severe head injury; in the other case the patient stopped breathing after rupture of a brain abscess. Both patients remained unconscious throughout artificial respiration and both ultimately died.

Respiration was measured by applying tightly a full face mask equipped with flutter valves; the air breathed out was conducted through a meter and measured. In both patients a tube was passed down through the larynx to insure an open airway. The blood was also analyzed for its gas contents and acidity.

In both cases the Schafer method of artificial respiration was almost completely inadequate. Two experienced operators were used in the administration of artificial respiration by this method, but the tidal air produced varied from about 72 to 117 cc. as compared to the normal value of 400 to 500 cc. On the other hand, the Eve tilting or gravity technic (described in the 1945 *Health Instruction Yearbook)* produced an adequate exchange of 286 to 500 cc. per cycle. The minute volume of air by the Schafer method ranged from 1,000 to 2,000 cubic centimeters, compared to a range of 4,000 to 6,000 cc. for the Eve method of artificial respiration.

The Schafer method depends to a large extent on the elastic recoil of the lungs and tone of the respiratory muscles, but *since these are absent in the deeply asphyxiated person, Schafer's method becomes of least value when most needed.* Conversely the Eve tilting method is efficient when tonus and elasticity of these structures are absent.

There are two important considerations in any discussion of artificial respiration. *The first is the time element. It is essential that the most immediately available method be used at once.* The second important consideration is that, as soon as possible, *the most efficient available method of artificial respiration should* replace the emergency measure.

foreign bodies in air passages

Hollinger, Paul H. *"Foreign Bodies in the Air and Food Passages," Transactions, American Academy of Ophthalmology and Otolaryngology, 66: 193-210, (No. 2), March-April, 1962.*

Paul H. Hollinger, M.D. reports on a review of 2,885 patients who were treated for removal of foreign bodies in the air or food passages over a period of 25 years.

Bone and meat particles, nut and vegetable objects, coins, discs, metallic objects and safety pins accounted for approximately 90 per cent of all the objects swallowed or aspirated in the last 500 cases. Major factors involved were hasty or gluttonous eating, laughing while eating, the use of dentures that made chewing difficult and disturbance of the swallowing mechanism by senility or alcohol.

Safety pins as foreign bodies are commonest in infants of diaper age. When safety pins are closed they do little harm and usually pass through the gastro-intestinal tract without lodging at any one point. A common story is that the mother pins the safety pin loosely to her dress while changing the infant's diaper and the pin falls into the baby's open mouth while he is crying. Long-standing disease of the esophagus, lungs or other parts of the body are sometimes traced to the unsuspected swallowing of an open safety pin during infancy. Sometimes older brothers or sisters feed the infant a foreign body.

One infant had four open safety pins in the esophagus. Often the baby will swallow a thumb tack that has been used to attach lace to a bassinet but falls into his open mouth.

Dried beans (from bean blowers) represent an urgent emergency even if the child is in good condition. When they are aspirated into a major bronchus, the absorption of moisture finally bursts the capsule of the bean and asphyxia may develop rapidly as the bean swells enough to block the trachea.

It seems incredible that razor blades can be chewed and swallowed, but five persons in this series did so. One adult swallowed three Schick blades that passed through spontaneously. One person attempted suicide but wrapped the blade in cellophane first. All five patients recovered.

The total deaths in the entire series amounted to only 0.3 per cent, or eight deaths in 2885 cases. Of this number five were infants and children and three of these infant deaths resulted from an open safety pin.

The treatment for foreign bodies has been influenced by modern techniques of anesthesia, radiology and chest surgery. A foreign body is not an emergency unless the airway is obstructed.

breath-holding spells in children

Linder, Charles W. "Breath-Holding Spells in Children," Clinical Pediatrics, 7: 88-90 (No. 2), February 1968.

A physician of Fitzsimons General Hospital in Denver, Colorado observes that the first good medical description of breath-holding was reported in 1848.

In this *study of 697 children* between the *ages of 6 months and 4 years* who were attending the pediatric clinic at the hospital, it was found that approximately *94 per cent had no history of breath-holding spells.* Of the children with breath-holding spells there were only 12 (less than 2 percent of the total) who had severe spells, while 33 others had mild ones.

In a second phase of the *study 20 children with severe breath-holding behaviors* were investigated more fully. The group was almost equally divided between boys and girls. The age of onset of the first breath-holding ranged from 3 to 17 months, but the average was approximately 10 months. *Within one year of follow-up study by* the physician 8 of the 20 children no longer had spells, and two were lost to the study. The eight children who had stopped did so after having an average of about one breath-holding episode per week. The range among those who had stopped, however, was from four per day to only one per month.

The children with severe breath-holding spells had similar personalities. They were *active, energetic, intelligent and independent.* They were thought to be more difficult to train and responded poorly to discipline. *Many were described by their parents as "nervous children." It often seemed to the examining physician that one or more of the parents had the same personality traits as the child.*

Most of the children in this investigation were physically normal, with no apparent organic causes of the spells. In 17 children studied with brain wave recordings, *six were found to have disturbances of rhythm suggestive of epilepsy,* yet when they were put on anticonvulsant treatment with phenobarbital, the spells were not completely controlled. With no medication whatsoever, some of the children ceased having their breath-holding episodes.

The best results were obtained by the reassurance given to parents and by improvements in the parent-child relationships.

The breath-holding spell can be distinguished from a convulsive seizure by careful observation. In breath-holding crying, cessation of breathing and bluish discoloration *precede* the loss the consciousness. In a convulsive seizure the cessation of breathing and bluish discoloration comes *after* the seizure, according to Dr. Linder.

tuberculosis from artificial respiration

Heilman, Kenneth M. and Carl Muschenheim. "Primary Cutaneous Tuberculosis Resulting from Mouth-to-Mouth Respiration," New England Journal of Medicine, 173: 1035-1036, November 4, 1965.

Two physicians from the Bellevue Hospital and the Cornell University Medical College of New York City report a case that illustrates the fact that *mouth-to-mouth breathing* or respiration *increases the chance of* the physician *developing tuberculosis.*

A 25-year old intern at Bellevue Hospital who had enjoyed good health throughout his entire life and who had a negative tuberculin skin test received a patient who was in a comatose condition and who shortly after admission to the hospital stopped breathing and had a cessation of heart beat. *In an attempt to save the life of the patient the young intern applied mouth-to-mouth respiration* and external cardiac massage. There was no reaction on the part of the patient to these life-saving measures and after five minutes the procedures were stopped and the patient was declared dead.

Six weeks after this experience a tuberculin skin test was repeated on the young physician because autopsy had revealed that the dead patient had active tuberculosis of the right lung. The skin test was strongly positive for the intern, although previously his skin test for tuberculosis had been negative.

About eight weeks after his attempt to revive the tuberculous patient the young intern observed a swollen lymph gland under the jaw and small pus-producing sores. Repeated cultures and examinations were needed before *it was finally proven that the intern had developed tuberculosis.* After twelve months of treatment with isoniazid (INH) each day, this antituberculosis drug was able to bring the disease under control and *no further evidence of the disease was noted.*

Most cases of tuberculosis of the skin have been found to occur in children and pathologists. This case is the first one reported as being due to mouth-to-mouth breathing.

Now at Bellevue Hospital the wards are equipped with rebreathing bags, tubes and other equipment that can be used instead of mouth-to-mouth respiration and the house staff has been trained in the use of this equipment. *It is hoped that with the use of this equipment that the need for mouth-to-mouth respiration will be reduced* and that the risks from this procedure will be reduced also.

4
drowning

Drowning and near-drowning are widely prevalent accidents, although they represent only part of the medical experience with the cessation of breathing. Drownings are not all the same, nor do some of the victims die from lack of oxygen alone, for there are many complicating factors that may threaten life in the near-drowning patient.

drowning

Miles, Stanley. "Drowning," British Medical Journal, 3: 597-600 (No. 5618), September 7, 1968.

A British physician of the Royal Naval Hospital in Plymouth reports that throughout the world *about 140,000 people are drowned each year.* The overcrowded islands of Japan, where much of the population is associated with fishing and aquatic sports, has the highest drowning rate in the world.

It is difficult to tell how many people actually lose their lives by drowning. A study in Great Britain, for example, showed that of 1,327 drowning deaths 290 were actually suicides.

The term "drowning" should be used when there is loss of consciousness and threat to life from submersion in water. When drowning results in death *the term "drowned"* should be used. *The term "secondary drowning"* should be used when the victim has apparently recovered from his drowning but loses his life due to later complications.

Ninety per cent of the people are buoyant enough to remain on the surface in fresh water with a small area of the scalp exposed, if they take a full breath. However, about 10 per cent will sink due to lack of buoyancy.

Dry drowning occurs in 20 to 40 per cent of all drowning cases.

When water enters the mouth it is swallowed in large amounts, but spasm of the larynx (upper part of the respiratory tract) may be so severe that all water is blocked from entering the lungs. Under such conditions neither can air enter the lungs, hence a person can lose consciousness without water entering the lungs. Dry drowning has the highest recovery rate if the victim can be rescued from the water.

Wet drowning involves the inhalation of water into the lungs. If inhalation of water occurs before loss of consciousness the victim may experience a severe and agonizing pain down the middle line of the chest. The entry of water into the lungs, fresh or salt, diminishes the oxygen-absorbing area of the lungs and disturbs the degree of electrolyte transfer (exchange of compounds in solution that conduct electricity). In all such cases there is a marked loss of protein from the blood, a factor that is involved in foam production. The characteristic foam that is found in the lungs and respiratory passages thus occurs because of the disturbance in the normal flow of electrolytes and the loss of blood protein.

Fresh water drowning usually involves circumstances different from those of salt water drowning. Fresh water has less buoyancy than salt water and drownings in the former tend to occur when the victim is alone (they are frequently suicidal). Also there is greater likelihood of entanglement in weeds or other underwater obstructions in fresh water. In most cases of fresh water drowning the water inhaled contains small marine growths, sand, mud, fuel oil, sewage or other pollutions that increase the hazard to the lungs. Often the drowning victim may appear to have recovered, but he may worsen rapidly with death occurring after respiratory distress, restlessness, pain in the chest, bluish discoloration of the skin, cough and the coughing or spitting of blood.

some facts about drowning

Staff. "Drowning," *Spectrum, 14: 66-68, (No. 3), Summer, 1966.*

New research and knowledge on the physiology of drowning or immersion may help to save lives. At the present time *about 7,000 persons* die from drowning each year in the United States. Many of the drowning victims are skin or scuba divers who are untrained, overconfident, careless, unlucky or physically or emotionally unfit for their sport.

One cause of drowning that was not suspected until recently is that of deep breathing before underwater swimming. Research has shown that over-breathing in an effort to enrich the blood with oxygen actually depletes the blood of carbon dioxide. The low level of carbon dioxide decreases the flow of blood through the brain, removes the urge to surface for the breathing-in of oxygen, and often results in unconsciousness which may result in drowning. No preliminary symptoms of an oxygen deficiency are apparent to the underwater swimmer under these circumstances. Practical considerations suggest that *no underwater swimmer should engage in deep breathing or over-breathing before he plunges under the water.*

Swimmers who dive repeatedly at brief intervals will progressively lower oxygen pressure in their lungs, even if they stay under water for no more than 30 seconds, and resurface for the same length of time before the next plunge. The oxygen supply to the brain is diminished and some subjects have suffered effects after only a few such dives.

It is commonly thought that the drowning man breathes water into his lungs, but in most drownings, spasm of the larynx prevents water from entering the lungs until the lack of oxygen becomes profound. Water is often swallowed in great amounts and is sometimes vomited and aspirated (breathed into the lungs). The lack of oxygen may cause convulsions, high blood pressure, vomiting, urination, defecation and coma, shock or death from respiratory and cardiac arrest.

It has been said often that the blood is diluted in fresh water drownings and concentrated in salt water drownings. The dilution of the blood may be associated with fibrillation of the heart and death, but research shows that in experimental animals who survive near-drowning, the blood rapidly regains a more normal concentration. Ultimately, a person drowned in either fresh or salt water has an increased concentration of the blood rather than a dilution.

Death in the drowning person results from stopping of the heart due to a lack of oxygen. The individual cells of the lungs are invaded by blood plasma, swelling, hemorrhage and destruction of blood cells due to the swelling, distension and rupture of the blood capillaries in the lung tissues. If death is delayed, inflammation of the lungs, pneumonia, and abscess may complicate recovery. *Whether death occurs early or late in drowning, it occurs from swelling of the lung tissues and a deficiency of oxygen to the brain.*

Attempts to drain water from the lungs are simply a waste of precious time. The immediate effort should be to restore respiration immediately. Mouth-to-mouth breathing can be accomplished even in the water. An important thing is to keep the airway open by looking to see that there is no debris in the throat and by keeping the head in extension to prevent the tongue from blocking the throat. The rescuer must concentrate on supplying air to the drowning victim.

The heart will not have stopped in most victims who can be saved, but if no evidence of heart action can be found, then external cardiac massage should be begun promptly in conjunction with the artificial respiration. Apparently hopeless cases have been saved even after 30 minutes by the combined use of these two methods of resuscitation. It is impossible to say with certainty exactly when death has occurred, and first aid measures should be continued while the patient is being transported to the hospital.

In the hospital the physician can be expected to use the administration of *oxygen, suction* from the throat and lung passages, *a mist or aerosol* to dilate the bronchial tubes leading to the lungs, rapid-acting *digitalis* to assist the heart and other measures to help in the restoration of normal heart action. Sometimes *blood plasma* may be needed. *Antibiotics* may be advisable if the victim has been in polluted water. Mineral *(electrolyte) balances* of the blood may be restored and a *lowering of body temperature* is generally considered advisable. The drowning victim must be watched carefully for 24 hours because the effects of drowning may be progressive even after apparent improvement.

When anyone is floundering in the water, it is prudent not to grapple with him because his desperation will have released epinephrine (adrenalin) to augment his strength, but not his sanity or judgment. It is best to give him a pole or rope.

Because of its buoyancy, the body does not submerge completely even when no effort is made to stay afloat. A technique based on this fact is known as *"drownproofing." All boaters and swimmers should learn it.* After taking a breath, the swimmer passively permits himself to sink below the water to his "natural" level, which is usually about the level of the eyebrows. Then he resurfaces in 8 to 10 seconds, exhales, and repeats the sinking process. This procedure can be continued for at least as long as six hours without fatigue or circulatory or respiratory difficulties.

One of the most extraordinary cases on record is that of a Norwegian boy of 5 years who was submerged in an icy river for more than 20 minutes. He was rescued by a policeman who used mouth-to-mouth breathing and cardiac massage. In the hospital for 24 hours the same procedures were used. The boy also received a blood transfusion, hydrocortisone, heart stimulants, and antibiotics. The patient was unconscious for six weeks, except for a brief period on the 10th day. Finally, when he was discharged from the hospital he appeared normal, except for some deterioration in vision and clumsiness in fine finger movements. [No comment is made on the possible damage to intelligence.—Ed.]

care of the near-drowning victim

Courington, Frederick W. and E. Warner Ahlgren. "Treatment of the Near-Drowning Victim," Texas Medicine, 65: 32-38, (No. 8), August 1969.

Two physicians, one with the U.S. Navy and the other with the University of Texas Southwestern Medical School in Dallas, Texas observe that *the care of the near-drowning victim has changed* within the last two or three years.

Emphasis in treatment has shifted to breathing, oxygen, circulation and acidosis.

In no instance should an effort be made to drain water from the patient's lungs; such efforts waste time and are fruitless. The airway must be cleared and breathing must be evaluated.

If the pulse rate or blood pressure is feeble or cannot be determined, external cardiac compression should be applied and continued until circulation of the blood is reestablished. The physician may also need to apply stimulants or tonics for the heart as well as oxygen as described in the foregoing paragraph.

Acidosis is an almost constant feature of the near-drowning victim. A lack of oxygen at the cell level occurs because of impairment of the circulation of the blood due to a reduction of output by the heart. This acidosis that involves the metabolism of the cells must be countered in the emergency room of the hospital by the administration of sodium bicarbonate.

The addition of sodium bicarbonate and oxygen are refinements in the emergency care of the near-drowning victim which must be provided in the hospital immediately after the patient arrives.

A decreased amount of oxygen in the tissues and organs of the body almost always leads to *vomiting* by the patient. He must be protected against aspiration of the vomitus. *Loss of body heat* is frequently evident and gradual warming is advisable.

For emergency care of the near-drowning victim the first aider should: 1) establish and maintain *a clear airway* (so the patient can breathe); 2) begin *mouth-to-mouth breathing;* 3) begin external cardiac massage if necessary; 4) summon *an emergency vehicle* for transportation to a hospital and 5) give *100 per cent oxygen if possible.* He *should not attempt to drain water* from the victim and he *should not slacken his efforts to save the victim for even a few seconds.*

an analysis of 163 drowning accidents

Adams, Anthony I. *"The Descriptive Epidemiology of Drowning Accidents," The Medical Journal of Australia, II: 1257-61, (No. 27), December 31, 1966.*

Anthony I. Adams, of the Department of Preventive Medicine at the University of Sydney in Sydney, Australia, reports on *163 drowning accidents* that occurred in the County of Cumberland, New South Wales, over a three-year period (January 1, 1962 to December 31, 1964.)

The pattern that emerges demonstrates a *high mortality among infants and young children,* a *marked lack of swimming ability in the majority of the victims,* a failure in many instances to appreciate the inherent danger of the situation, or gross *foolhardiness or negligence* prior to the accident.

Of the 163 persons drowned, 137 were males and 26 were females. Most of the accidents (44) were associated with swimming. Surfing claimed 10 lives, 9 persons were washed off rocks while fishing, 24 drowned following boating mishaps, one while water skiing, and three while skin diving. Nineteen drowned when doing nothing more than standing near the water and falling in, often as a result of alcoholic intoxication or a medical condition such as epilepsy or heart attack. Thirty-eight children drowned while playing near water (28 of these were under four years of age), and 15 drowned in baths.

The majority of accidents occurred in the *warmer months* of the year, on *weekends,* and between *midday and 3 p.m.* Fifty-seven persons drowned in the ocean, 45 in rivers, 21 in swimming pools, 16 in or around a bath, 10 in ponds or dams, six in lakes, one in a canal, and seven in various other situations.

The outcome of an accident involving submersion is influenced by a number of factors such as environmental conditions and the person's health and physical condition; but of greatest importance is his ability to stay afloat and perhaps swim some distance, plus the availability of assistance in the form of other people nearby.

Forty-five per cent of the total were alone at the time of the tragedy, 18 per cent had one companion, 15 per cent had two companions, and 22 per cent were accompanied by more than two others. Of those over five years of age, 39 per cent were non-swimmers, 39 per cent were average swimmers, and 22 per cent were excellent swimmers.

Of the 163 drowned, 128 were in good health. The remaining *35 had various ailments,* including heart disease, epilepsy, diabetes, and other pre-existing conditions. *In 25 of these cases, it was concluded that the main cause of loss of life from drowning was related to the victim's impaired state of health.*

Twenty-two of the 163 victims were said to be intoxicated at the time of the accident, but *the actual figure is probably higher* than that. Under the influence of alcohol, judgment is impaired and physical stamina rapidly wanes. *Alcohol appears to be a significant factor in drowning accidents* as well as in traffic accidents.

An attempt was made to classify the 163 fatalities by what appeared to be the *major factors* in their causation. Sixty-three people (39 per cent) drowned due to *foolhardy or irresponsible action* by themselves or others. Included are non-swimmers who went into deep water or went out alone in small boats, persons using underwater diving equipment without any previous experience, persons attempting water sports while intoxicated, persons surfing at night or in rough seas on unpatrolled beaches, and persons fishing off cliffs in obviously perilous circumstances.

Thirty-nine (24 per cent) drowned through the *failure of their guardians to provide adequate supervision.* Most of these were babies or young children left alone in their baths or left unattended to roam in the vicinity of water.

Twenty-five (15 per cent) drowned as a result of some *incapacitating medical condition,* and 23 (14 per cent) died as a result of *danger-*

ous environmental factors. To the remaining 13 fatalities (8 per cent), no major cause could be assigned.

The *high percentage of non-swimmers* among those drowned—86 per cent of those aged five to nine years, 50 per cent of those aged 10 to 14 years, and 25 per cent of those aged 15 to 24 years—demands attention. All children over the age of five years should be able to swim at least 25 yards and stay afloat for an indefinite period in calm water.

Another impressing fact is that *most people have little idea of the potential danger* in which they so often place themselves or others. More warning notices in certain places might be of some value, but many of these drowning accidents occurred in places where signs and notices were already present warning of unsafe conditions. *Water, like the motor vehicle, should not be underestimated as a threat to life.*

The following actions, if taken, could help in reducing the number of drowning deaths that occur each year:

(1) No baby should be left unattended in its bath.

(2) No child under the age of five years, or small child who cannot swim, should be left alone without adult supervision in or *near water.*

(3) All backyard or neighborhood swimming pools, fish ponds, dams, canals and tanks should be child-proof. Private swimming pools should be emptied during winter.

(4) Everyone over the age of five years should be taught to swim.

(5) Non-swimmers or persons subject to epileptic fits should not go out in small boats or engage in any water sport unaccompanied.

(6) The hazards involved when amateurs engage in rock fishing, boating, and underwater diving should be made more widely known.

(7) The consumption of alcohol by anyone engaged in any form of activity relating to water should be limited.

5
bleeding

External hemorrhage is one of the critical conditions in first aid if it is severe in nature. It is also one of the emergencies most responsive to proper first aid care, for the application of a simple, direct compress at the bleeding point is a procedure that most anyone can follow.

There are many aspects to bleeding problems other than injuries that produce them. Most of this information can be found only in the medical literature. This chapter is only a brief introduction to the subject.

bleeding disorders

Goulian, Mehran. "A Guide to Disorders of Hemostasis," Annals of Internal Medicine, 65: 782-796, (No. 4), October 1966.

A physician from the Department of Medicine of the Harvard Medical School and the Massachusetts General Hospital in Boston reports that recent *advances have been made in the scientific understanding of hemorrhage* and its control.

There are *four areas into which bleeding disorders can be classified* in terms of their involvement: 1) the *blood vessels;* 2) the *platelets* of the blood; 3) the *coagulation or clotting process* itself; and 4) *stability of the clot* after it has been formed.

The blood vessels may be involved in bleeding because of abnormalities in the vessels or in the supporting tissues around them. The vessels may have extreme fragility or defective contractility. Such defects of structure or function may be hereditary in origin. An example is a bleeding disease known as hereditary hemorrhagic telangiectasia.

Blood platelets appear to have two different functions in the control of bleeding. The first is associated with the coagulation of blood (the clotting process) and the second is concerned with the integrity of the small blood vessels. In the latter the function of the platelets is not clear, but the platelets may be involved in plugging small breaks or rents in the small blood vessels. Whenever the platelets do not function properly in preserving the integrity of the small blood vessels, blood emerges beneath the skin to form small hemorrhages and purple patches on the skin.

Coagulation, or the clotting process, may be involved in bleeding diseases or the control of bleeding. *Ten different clotting factors* have now been identified by scientists and have been given Roman numerals. Fibrinogen and prothrombin (I and II) are still commonly identified by their old names. Coagulation occurs in definite steps, but the full process is not completely clear. The formation of fibrin appears to occur at the end stage of a sequence of events. *Clot stability or instability* may be involved in some bleeding diseases. The clot may be formed, but it is defective or else it is destroyed by the action of substances in the blood. The clot-dissolving system may act directly on the clot, or indirectly on clotting factors in the blood.

Disorders in the control of bleeding may be due to heredity or to some acquired factor. Hemophilia A (Factor VIII deficiency) makes up about 80 per cent of all hereditary bleeding disorders. It is inherited as a sex-linked recessive that affects males and is transmitted by females, who are usually unaffected. All gradations of the disease occur and in mild hemophilia there may be little or no abnormal bleeding. *Acquired factors* may involve the platelets, liver disease, Vitamin K deficiency, abnormal blood vessels, anticoagulants that circulate in the blood and other factors.

bleeding in head injury

Abbott, Kenneth H. "Acute Intracranial Epidural Hemorrhage," Ohio State Medical Journal, 51: 666-68 (No. 7), July 1955.

Kenneth H. Abbott, M.D., Assistant Professor of Neurosurgery at the Ohio State University College of Medicine, points out that an acute intracranial epidural hemorrhage is frequently a serious complication of any head injury of apparent mild or serious degree.

An epidural hemorrhage is one that occurs between the skull and the lining of the brain. *This type of hemorrhage should be suspected when the head injury has resulted in loss of consciousness.* This primary loss of consciousness may be for a relatively short time and may be expressed in seconds or minutes or possibly a little longer.

After the person who has suffered the head injury has regained consciousness there may be no symptoms and the patient may appear to be subjectively normal or with only minor complaints of headache. It is during this second phase that the blood is accumulating in the epidural space. As the clot increases in size, brain compression and deformity take place, and the patient becomes confused and lethargic until unconsciousness intervenes. Paralysis, pupillary changes, and convulsions may or may not be present, and when present are probably not of localizing (lateralizing) value in over 50 per cent of the cases.

The entire series of signs and symptoms may occur in the course of a few hours, or even within an hour or less. Less commonly this may take place over a period of days. *When the patient reaches the stage where he is getting confused and lethargic there is very little time left for the prevention of permanent damage or the saving of life.*

The absence of fracture is no guarantee that there is not a blood clot present, although the presence of a fracture line should be taken as a helpful sign of suspicion of the presence of a clot, provided some other sign of cerebral compression is present or beginning to appear.

If the surgeon suspects the presence of an epidural clot, it is then necessary that immediate surgery be embarked upon at the earliest possible moment. This is an acute emergency, just as is the case of an external hemorrhage from a major blood vessel.

Sometimes there may be no primary period of loss of consciousness and the blood may accumulate very slowly in the epidural space with slow development of symptoms such as headache, nausea, vomiting, double vision, unequal pupils, convulsions, and paralysis. This may last from hours to days and has been known to last for several weeks.

Eventually this slow type of hemorrhage is followed by the gradual or rapid development of coma and death with respiratory failure first.

In small infants the brain may accommodate fairly large blood clots in the epidural space for unusually long times, probably because of the ability of the brain to withstand distortion. The same situation may occur in the aged, when extensive cerebral atrophy is present, thus allowing space for large blood clots to develop before any serious compression of the brain occurs.

symptoms and signs of brain hemorrhage

Calvert, James M. "Premonitory Symptoms and Signs of Subarachnoid Hemorrhage," Medical Journal of Australia, 1: 651-57 (No. 16), April 16, 1966.

A physician from the Department of Neurosurgery at the Alfred Hospital in Melbourne, Australia, reports on *200 cases of hemorrhage occurring under the middle layer of the brain.* The majority of these hemorrhages were caused by the rupture of a blood-containing bulge on an artery (aneurysm) or a similar type of blood-filled swelling or tumor in the brain.

The onset of symptoms was sudden and dramatic in most cases, without previous warning. However, in an appreciable number of cases, questioning of the patient after the acute stage had passed revealed *a pattern of symptoms* which, had they been reported to a physician, might have led to preventive treatment before the actual hemorrhage, with its often disastrous consequences, had occurred.

Headache (non-migraine) was the most frequent symptom preceding hemorrhage, and occurred in 63 of the 200 cases. Another 6 patients had suffered from headache of the migraine type. It is probable that many aneurysms, prior to complete rupture, have one or more slight leakages of blood, so that there may be episodes of acute headaches, often accompanied by *neck stiffness.*

Pressure caused by the aneurysm may affect the nerves and muscles of the eye. Other important symptoms which may occur prior to hemorrhage are *drooping of an eyelid, squinting, a dilated pupil in one eye,* or *double vision.* These signs are indicative of expansion of the aneurysm and are important warning signs of its impending rupture.

Other less-common warning signs reported by some of the patients included *convulsions, mental changes* (deterioration of memory and concentration, lethargy, blunted intellect), *disturbances of consciousness, speech, sensation, and motor power, visual field disturbances, dizziness,* and general *malaise* (especially nausea). A surprising number of patients gave a *history of a "stroke"* occurring several years previously, for which they had been treated only by bed rest with no investigation of cause. Occasionally there was a striking *family history* of known aneurysms, or of early death from "brain hemorrhage."

Although many people have aneurysms which never cause any trouble, symptoms which increase in frequency and severity can be regarded as warning of impending rupture. It is important to diagnose and treat an aneurysm before rupture; probably at least 60 per cent of patients die from the first or recurrent hemorrhages, and another 20 per cent are incapacitated.

emergency care of injury to blood vessels

Herrmann, Louis G. "Management of Injuries to Large Blood Vessels in Wounds of Violence," The American Journal of Surgery, 74: 560-75, (No. 5), November 1947.

Louis G. Herrmann, M.D., of the Department of Surgery, College of Medicine, at the University of Cincinnati, says that *the immediate seriousness of wounds of violence depends to a great degree upon the extent and kind of injury to the underlying blood vessels.*

The muscles of an arm or leg may undergo tissue death in six to ten hours if the extremity is deprived of an adequate arterial circulation. In most wounds of violence which affect the extremities, there is also considerable damage to the surrounding tissues, especially the nerves, and frequently to the bones. Often there is severe shock associated with these injuries, resulting from loss of blood volume with a fall of blood pressure.

The immediate treatment of any injury which involves large blood vessels must be directed toward the prevention of excessive loss of blood. *The application of a tourniquet above the site of the injury to control bleeding must be discouraged since such a measure deprives the entire extremity of arterial blood.* Even after a relatively short period of time, the lack of oxygen may produce irreparable damage to the soft tissues. When hemorrhage is less severe and there is the possibility of preserving the limb, *the bleeding should be arrested by finger compression over the wound, followed by compression bandages.* The wound can then be packed with gauze and a reasonable amount of pressure can be applied through the bandage until the bleeding is completely stopped.

In addition to the direct attack upon the bleeding vessels, there are other valuable methods of diminishing the rate and amount of bleeding. *With vertical elevation of the extremities and mild direct pressure in the wound the bleeding from almost any peripheral artery can be controlled temporarily. Vertical elevation alone often suffices to stop the bleeding from a lacerated artery of the forearm, leg, or foot.*

proper use of the tourniquet

Wolff, Luther H., and Trogler F. Adams. "Tourniquet Problems in War Injuries," Bulletin of the United States Army Medical Department, pp. 77-84, (No. 87), April 1945.

Major Luther H. Wolff and Captain Trogler F. Adams, of the United States Army Medical Corps, reported from their experience on the Italian war front that the intelligent handling of tourniquets in war injuries of the extremities has been considerably neglected. The whole tourniquet question too often has been lightheartedly dismissed with the suggestion, "Release tourniquets every twenty minutes to one-half hour," whereas *the problem requires thought and sound judgment. Tourniquets are frequently applied unnecessarily, but the rule of releasing tourniquets every one-half hour to "prevent gangrene" is extremely dangerous in many instances.*

1 *An adequate tourniquet.* Complete control of bleeding is the primary aim of tourniquet application, and any procedure short of this is considered inadequate. The strap-and-buckle tourniquet is too narrow and cuts into the tissues, and it rarely completely controls bleeding no matter how tightly applied.
The simplest and most effective device for a tourniquet is one of soft rubber tubing properly applied. This tubing should be at least six feet long. A good procedure is to pad the extremity with a towel, a shirt sleeve, trouser leg, or any other material available, at the level at which the tourniquet is to be applied. Four parallel turns of the rubber tubing are wound around the leg under moderate tension only, the end first applied being overlapped and anchored by the second turn, and the last turn being anchored by the next to the last turn. *Most rubber-tubing tourniquets are applied too tightly;* actually, if several turns are used, only moderate tension is required to occlude all vessels completely.
A tourniquet should be placed as close to the site of injury in the thigh or arm as is feasible. If large defects are present in the extremity, care must be taken that the tourniquet is placed sufficiently above the injury to prevent the tourniquet from slipping down into the defect.

2 *When to apply a tourniquet.* Many severe wounds of extremities not involving major blood vessels require no tourniquet. An inadequate tourniquet may actually increase bleeding from this type of wound. Yet the impression gained on the Italian battle front was that tourniquets have not been used sufficiently nor early enough in serious extremity wounds, particularly in wounds involving large blood vessels or inpatients with amputations. Statistics are not available to show what percentage of wounded bleed to death on the battlefield

from extremity wounds, nor is it known how many succumb from hemorrhage after receiving first-aid treatment. It seems probable that some do, although the proportion may be small.
Spontaneous arrest of hemorrhage frequently does not take place until the blood pressure has fallen and sufficient spasm has developed in the vessels to effect cessation of flow. This is a somewhat dangerous method to rely on to control hemorrhage.

3 *The time factor.* Fear of possible damage to an extremity from a tourniquet seems based on no reasonable grounds. The greatest fear is exhibited regarding "gangrene" of an extremity. Unquestionably an extremity will become gangrenous if a tourniquet is left on an excessive length of time; but a tourniquet may be left on for from two to six hours, depending on the temperature of the atmosphere and of the extremity, without detectable damage. Tourniquets have been left on as long as eight hours, during the winter of 1943-44, without apparent harmful effect. Tourniquets applied for four to six hours without loosening have been observed on several occasions. Surgeons of an auxiliary surgical group performed amputations on about 1,000 patients in forward hospitals. These surgeons have all seen extremities on which tourniquets have been left applied up to four hours; yet no case of gangrene solely from a tourniquet has been noted. In a temperate climate a tourniquet left in place for a period of from two to four hours causes no particular harm from depriving the tissues of circulation. The fear of producing tourniquet gangrene unless the tourniquet is loosened every half hour seems baseless.

4 *The tourniquet in relation to patients in shock.* There are cases in which the removal or loosening of a tourniquet is unwise and unnecessary; in fact, the results may be disastrous. *Under no circumstances should a tourniquet be loosened on a patient in shock or in incipient shock unless means are present and immediately available to control hemorrhage and to replace rapidly the volume of circulating blood.*
It is true that an individual who has lost a moderate amount of blood can tolerate additional, mild, rapid loss of blood without his recovery

being jeopardized in the least. There are many patients, however, who have lost blood up to their critical level. In these individuals the most urgent care must be used to prevent additional loss of blood volume. The rapid loss of even a small amount of blood may completely break down the delicately balanced mechanism so that the vasoconstricting apparatus fails, with resultant profound, and possibly irreversible, shock. In such instances it is safe to loosen an applied tourniquet only after the blood volume has been brought up to some extent by plasma or, preferably, by whole-blood transfusions.

Patients may lose more blood than is first apparent on loosening a tourniquet, particularly in the thigh. The arterial system fills up more or less uniformly on the release of a tourniquet, and if the vascular injury is some distance below the tourniquet the injured area will continue to drain off this blood, even though the blood supply is shut off promptly at the first sign of hemorrhage.

5 *The temperature factor.* Temperature has been shown by experimental workers to play a vital part in the speed with which death of a bloodless extremity takes place. *The metabolic demands of tissues of a bloodless extremity vary directly with its temperature.* A cold extremity survives longer than a warm extremity when a tourniquet is applied. In general, therefore, a tourniquet applied in the heat of the tropics or of the desert should be loosened at shorter intervals than one applied in a cool climate. It is suggested that an extremity on which a tourniquet has been placed should be left uncovered, and that no attempt made to warm the extremity by artificial means until the tourniquet is ready to be removed—care being used, of course, to prevent frostbite in sub-freezing weather.

basic mechanisms in nosebleed

Jacobson, Philip. "The Mechanism of Epistaxis," Virginia Medical Monthly 93: 197-208, (No. 4), April 1966.
A physician of Petersburg, Virginia reports that from his studies and observations on nosebleed (epistaxis) that it is the most common form of spontaneous hemorrhage.

This physician believes that *nosebleed represents an inherent bleeding mechanism* that can strike anywhere in the body and can be a menace throughout life.

In his studies of nosebleed Dr. Jacobson asked himself such questions as the following: how does so much blood escape when there are no vessels capable of carrying so much blood in the nose? how is the blood released? does the blood escape passively or is it actively expelled? what becomes of the bleeding point and how does it disappear so rapidly?

Dr. Jacobson's studies so far support the view that *damage to the nasal mucosa disappears rapidly* because congestion of nasal tissues is reduced within minutes and regeneration of the nasal epithelium requires only a few hours.

Spontaneous hemorrhages occur so often throughout the body that every branch of medicine must contend with this problem. Such hemorrhages, according to Dr. Jacobson, are comparable to epistaxis. He reports three cases of nosebleed associated with different diseases in which each of the patients died. Although they died of different diseases, nosebleed was a common factor. A patient with rheumatic fever bled from both sides of the nose; one who died from nephritis (kidney disease) had a sudden explosive hemorrhage from the left side of the nasal septum. The third victim did not bleed from the septum at all, but only from the nasal turbinates. Grossly, *the bleeding surfaces were congested, but there were no open vessels.* A special search was made for exits for the blood. No openings were found that were large enough for the amount of blood involved. Dr. Jacobson concluded that blood does not escape passively, but that it is expelled. The mechanism for the process is not clear, but Dr. Jacobson believes that a deficiency of estrogens is involved and that the action is on the blood vessels rather than on the overlying epithelium, as some investigators believe.

This physician believes that the mechanism of nosebleed extends far beyond just having a nosebleed. Many investigators have noted a relationship between bleeding from hemorrhoids, hemorrhages under the skin, and the bleeding from pulmonary tuberculosis, all of which *can be helped by the intravenous injection of estrogen.*

Dr. Jacobson believes that the *diverse examples of spontaneous bleeding must be started by an inherent stimulus connected with the endocrine system,* unless the hemorrhage is from such a large vessel that measures other than estrogen treatment are needed.

No patient bleeds all of the time. The bleeding occurs in episodes with irregular intervals in between. Accident or injury seldom starts the bleeding because the points of injury are surrounded by walls of bone and hidden by deviations in the septum.

Previous episodes of bleeding are not the marks of a bleeder, but it should be a warning that complications are more likely than if there were no such history.

How seepage through the blood vessels can occur is not clear. There must be at least three actions in this process: an increase in blood pressure; loss of contractility of the blood vessel and greater permeability of the walls of the blood vessel.

According to Dr. Jacobson, *estrogen does not control nosebleed by the acceleration of coagulation. There are no open vessels to be sealed by a clot,* and even if there were, the clotting agents would be washed away. Estrogen treatment appears to be a replacement treatment in which the action is upon the walls of the blood vessels.

nosebleed

Staff. *"Epistaxis," Spectrum 14: 16-17, (No. 1), Winter 1965-1966.*

Most nosebleeds are minor and self-limited, but there is no way of knowing that any episode is not serious until after it has stopped. Persistent bleeding is a horrifying experience for both the bleeder and the physician who fails to control it. Since the physician is not likely to be called in until after there is just cause for alarm, he may have a serious problem on his hands.

The principles of first-aid treatment (before the doctor arrives) are virtually the same whether the bleeding is traumatic, infectious or spontaneous.

The patient should stand if possible, or at least sit up, in order to keep blood pressure in the nose at a minimum, and his head should be inclined forward so as to minimize the amount of blood swallowed. In some 90 per cent of the cases, the bleeding is in Little's area, the lower, forward third of the nasal septum, which abounds in capillaries. A plastic nose clamp may control it, or even a spring-type clothespin or simple pinching with the fingers.

Once the immediate episode is brought under control, diagnosis of the cause is essential to prevent recurrence. Diagnosis seldom presents a problem if the cause is an injury, but it may not do much good to advise a little boy to keep out of fist fights or an adult to avoid accidents. Some types of injury are more easily preventable, however, especially violent blowing of the nose, picking at it, or the childish habit of inserting foreign objects in the nose. If dry air is a factor, as it often is in centrally heated American houses, a humidifier can be recommended. Some patients should be advised to avoid contaminated air or high altitude insofar as possible. The vascular wall degenerates in a host of infections, such as scarlet and rheumatic fevers, whooping cough, measles, and smallpox.

Chronic bleeding may be an early manifestation of leprosy, and persistent bleeding from both nostrils can be grounds for suspecting nasal diphtheria. Vascular fragility and increased permeability are associated with various systemic diseases, including diabetes, allergies, scurvy or mild ascorbic acid deficiency, and the anemias. Salicylate, arsenic, mercury or phosphorus poisoning, excessive use of tobacco (especially snuff) or vasoconstrictors, and occasionally medication with antihistamines or barbiturates can damage the vascular wall. Such bleeding is recurrent but usually not persistent.

There are many other causes of nosebleed, such as high blood pressure, arteriosclerosis and other disorders.

6
shock

Shock is a most complicated phenomenon on which considerable research is being done, but which is still unexplained in many respects. There are many different causes of shock, all of which may threaten life. The most effective emergency handling and medical treatment of shock depends upon recognition of its cause as well as in the application of those general measures that apply to all cases.

Shock is such a difficult problem that the first aider needs to recognize that his greatest contribution to the victim may lie in swift access to medical and hospital services. First aid measures in some forms of shock, however, may make the difference between survival and death.

eight basic causes of shock

Rushmer, Robert F., Robert L. Van Citters and Dean L. Franklin. "Shock: A Semantic Enigma," Circulation, 26: 445-59, September 1962.

Two physicians and a physiologist from the University of Washington School of Medicine in Seattle observe that clarification of semantic confusion in the field of shock research is necessary.

"Shock" is a term used to describe the signs and symptoms associated with lowered blood pressure, a fast pulse, and a cold, pale skin of the face and extremities. The complex set of symptoms known as shock may arise from a wide assortment of causes, such as hemorrhage, injury, heart attack, peritonitis, anaphylaxis (allergic sensitivity) and other conditions. To be properly defined and understood, shock must be related to its cause.

The basic causes of shock can be found among the many different causes of a lowered arterial blood pressure.

1 *Loss of blood* (exsanguination). The average adult can lose about 500 ml. blood without significant disturbance. When the arterial blood pressure falls to 60 mm. Hg or lower, however, a shock condition exists and there is a need for restoration of blood volume.

2 *Loss of large amounts of body fluid* (deshydremia). In certain infectious diseases such as cholera, in severe burns, in water depletion and certain other conditions there may be great loss of body fluid with a reduction in the fluid part of the blood (plasma). Loss of plasma fluid into the tissues can produce the same result.

3 *Concentration or trapping of the blood in certain restricted parts of the circulatory system* (sequestration). Nearly 75 per cent of the total blood volume is in the venous system. If the capacity of some part of this system suddenly increased a substantial part of the blood supply could be sequestered and results corresponding to an external blood loss could be produced. During prolonged quiet standing, for example, greater than normal amounts of blood may accumulate in the veins of the legs and fainting may occur. Injury, peritonitis, and the crush syndrome may produce sequestration of the blood volume.

4 *Injury (trauma)*. The effects of injury may be widespread and diverse. Blood may escape into the tissues or outside the body; distention of the veins in injured parts may lead to sequestration, autonomic controls of the heart and peripheral vessels may be disturbed, and dilation of the injured vessels can lead to a reduction of peripheral resistance.

5 *Cardiac compression*. The collection of blood or other fluid in the sac around the heart (pericardial sac) can compress the latter so that its normal filling is restricted. Subsequently the heart is unable to deliver its normal capacity of blood with each stroke.

6 *Heart attack*. The rupture of a blood vessel in the heart itself reduces the volume of blood that the heart can deliver with each stroke. The damaged part of the heart cannot contract; this reduces the capacity for maintaining a normal cardiac output.

7 *Autonomic imbalance.* The sympathetic nervous system affects the stroke volume, the heart rate and the total resistance of the peripheral vessels. A severe depression of arterial blood pressure can result from autonomic imbalance. A slow heart beat and dilation of the blood vessels in certain regions of the body (e.g. skeletal muscle) are characteristic of autonomic imbalance. Head injury may produce a shock-like state through the mechanism of autonomic imbalance.

8 *Expansion of the peripheral blood vessels.* Shock may be caused by a fall in total peripheral resistance. Peritonitis, crush injury, and anaphylaxis are all characterized by extreme expansion of the blood vessels. An increased pulse and cardiac output are compensatory efforts of the body to sustain arterial pressure.

shock lung

Cline, Martin J., David Lehman, John F. Murray, Hibbard E. Williams and Lloyd H. Smith, Jr. "Shock Lung," *California Medicine*, 112: 43-50, (No. 2), February 1970.

A medical staff conference at the University of California Medical Center in San Francisco was concerned with *a newly understood kind of shock known as "shock lung."* In Vietnam battle casualties *the typical signs of "shock lung" included progressively more difficult breathing, progressive deficiency of oxygen, falling blood pressure, followed by 12 to 24 hours of freedom from respiratory abnormalities. After this period, however, there was increased shortness of breath and a progressive fall of oxygen in arterial blood. After death the lungs have been found to contain hemorrhages, to be congested and without air.* There is intense congestion and spaces are filled with fluid and blood. Blood clots and death of lung tissues are also evident.

Many factors are involved in "shock lung." Toxic or poisonous substances are known to result from infections, chemical substances, absorption from the intestines, and possible release of substances from devitalized or dead tissue during shock. *Many substances in the blood are also known to exert profound effects on the lung that can cause abnormal lung function.* During shock *clotting factors in the blood may* play an important role in producing "shock lung." *An extremely important* factor is over-hydration. In some battlefield patients gallons of fluid have been replaced by massive and swift action within 12 to 14 hours. Most patients in shock are given high concentrations of oxygen and it is thought that too much oxygen may produce toxic effects. *Infections* are involved in shock lung frequently because the normal capacity of the lung to remove harmful materials is often substantially impaired. The *small blood vessels of the lung* seem to be involved. For example, small blood clots plug the arteries and raise the blood pressure within the lungs. Congestion of the blood vessels in the lungs occurs and *blood leaks into the lungs.* Changes in the permeability of the blood vessels seem to be involved. *Substantially less oxygen* is picked up by the blood in the lung tissues because there is swelling and filling of the lungs with fluid. *The release of carbon dioxide* from the blood is impaired also because of the damage to the lungs. As shock lung increases the amount of carbon dioxide in the blood continues to rise. Because of the accumulation of fluid in the lungs the patient cannot tolerate injection of fluids by vein. *High concentrations of oxygen for 4 to 6 days seems to damage lung tissues* and create more problems.

From the experiments and clinical experience of the physicians in this conference it has been concluded that *respiratory failure, a frequent accompaniment of shock,* can occur in any patient and that multiple factors are involved. *The lack of oxygen* in the blood, the *inability of the lung to ventilate properly,* and other factors may be involved, such as *disturbances of blood clotting.*

shock from diminished blood volume

Baker, Robert J. and William C. Shoemaker. "Changing Concepts in Treatment of Hypovolemic Shock," Arizona Medicine, 26: 140-148, (No. 2), February 1969.

Two Chicago surgeons report that an enormous body of information on shock caused by a reduction of blood volume, such as from massive bleeding, has accumulated in the last 10 years.

Shock has been defined in many ways, but in essence, it refers to an inablility of the circulatory system to provide enough blood to the vital organs.

The most important vital organs in terms of decreasing importance are the brain, heart, lung, liver, and kidney. *If these organs are receiving an adequate supply of blood then the circulatory system is reasonably intact and shock has not occurred. Shock is a defect in the flow of blood through the tissues (tissue perfusion defect) rather than a defect of central pressure.*

Whenever there is a significant loss of blood volume (from 12 to 20 per cent or more) an extremely complex series of events is set into motion, an understanding of which is beyond most laymen. However, this new knowledge has changed some classic concepts of the treatment of shock. The treatment of a major blood loss is now known to require more than just the replacement of blood volume. Measures must be taken also to decrease the peripheral resistance, to increase the output of the heart and to provide support for the lung and kidney. In a man of about 150 pounds shock levels in relation to the loss of blood and clinical findings are described in the following table.

70 shock

Shock Level and Bleeding Category	Loss of Blood	Signs & Symptoms
A. Modest Bleeding (No shock)	15% of circulating blood volume (750 ml. or less)	Accelerated heart rate (pulse 112 or less) Cool skin Negative capillary blanching No postural disturbance Normal central venous pressure Normal hourly urine volume
B. Moderate Bleeding (Shock occurs late)	20 to 25% of circulating blood volume (1000 to 1250 ml.)	Accelerated heart rate (pulse 120) Cool, moist skin Decreased pulse pressure Positive capillary blanching Postural dizziness, fainting Low central venous pressure Borderline hourly urine volume
C. Advanced Bleeding (Admitted to hospital in shock)	30 to 35% of circulating blood volume (1500 to 1750 ml.)	Greatly accelerated heart rate Cold, clammy skin Pallor Hypotension Very low central venous pressure Hourly urine output very low (5 to 15 ml.)
D. Massive Bleeding	40 to 45% of circulating blood volume (2000 to 2250 ml.)	Profound shock Lethargy, stupor Diminished reflexes Zero or negative central venous pressure No urine output

shock and its effects on human cells

Schumer, William and Richard Sperling. "Shock and Its Effect on the Cell," Journal of the American Medical Association, 205: 215-219, (No. 4), July 22, 1968.

Two physicians from the Surgical Service of the University of Illinois College of Medicine in Chicago report that *new research on shock has* emphasized the treatment of the metabolism of the cell, in terms of its breakdown and repair during shock conditions.

Shock is a disease of the molecules. The disturbances of shock revolve around the metabolism of blood sugar (glucose). When there is low filtration of various normal substances through the individual cell walls due to shock conditions the metabolism of blood sugar under conditions within the cell *without adequate amounts of oxygen* (anaerobic conditions), is changed. There is an *increase within the cell of lactic acids, amino acids, fatty acids, and phosphoric acids.* This increase in acid conditions within the cell results in a rupture of the membranes of lysosomes with an outpouring of enzymes that causes the death of the cell. (Lysosomes are very small bodies that can be seen under the electron microscope in many types of cells. They contain various kinds of enzymes that can change many compounds through the addition of water).

As acid conditions develop within the cell the lysosomes rupture and release enzymes that increase the flow of water into the total cell and its individual parts. Under shock conditions *there is also a reduction of protein synthesis and a disturbance of the cell membrane* that causes sodium and water to flow into the cell and potassium to flow out of the cell. The sodium and water cause *swelling of the cell* and also of some of the contents of the cell. The result is the death of the cell.

The *treatment of shock that takes account of what is happening to the individual cells of the body would be as follows:*

1 *Replenishment of blood volume,* containing red blood cells that carry oxygen to the tissues.

2 *Energizing solutions are introduced* containing high concentrations of glucose (blood sugar), potassium, and insulin. These energizing solutions induce the blood sugar (glucose) to cross the cell membranes into the cell. As oxygen within the cells returns to normal, along with sugar concentrations, then normal cellular metabolism begins to be restored.

3 *Acids that have already formed are neutralized* by the use of antacids such as sodium bicarbonate or other substances. The lactic acid buildup in the cell is reversed.

4 *Corticoids* (hormones of the adrenal cortex or comparable synthetic compounds) *are given* to dilate blood vessels, increase amino acids and fats, convert lactic acid to glycogen and protect lysosomes.

bee sting and anaphylactic shock

Houser, D. Duane and Irvin Caplin. *"Insect-Sting Allergy," American Journal of Diseases of Children*, 113: 498-503, (No. 4), April 1967.

Two physicians from the Allergy Clinic of the Indiana University Medical School report that many unexplained, *sudden deaths* in the out-of-doors during the summer months *may be due to insect-sting allergy.*

The first recorded death from an insect sting was that of King Menes of Egypt, who died of a hornet sting in 2642 B.C. Four thousand years later a diagnosis of anaphylactic shock due to an allergic reaction was made by a modern physician.

In one medical review of deaths from venomous animals and insects covering a period of 10 years and 460 fatalities, it was found that stinging insects caused 220 of the deaths—far more than snake bites caused.

Bees, wasps, hornets and yellow jackets account for most of the deaths from stinging insects, in the order named.

Local swelling from a sting does not indicate an allergic reaction. A greater reaction is needed, such as urticaria (a hive-like swelling or wheal), generalized itching, nasal congestion, sneezing, asthma (difficulty in breathing), abdominal cramps, nausea and vomiting, swelling of the air passages in the throat or chest, difficulty in swallowing, circulatory collapse and death. The more severe reactions usually occur in less than 30 minutes. Occasionally a delayed serum-sickness-type of reaction may come on many hours or several days after an insect sting. Local reactions, however, are usually not allergic.

Sometimes it is difficult for the physician to distinguish between a reaction that is caused by a toxic (poisonous) reaction or a psychological reaction (with giddiness, overbreathing, gastrointestinal complaints and fainting) from a genuine allergic reaction. Because death may occur rapidly from an allergic reaction *it is safest to assume that a toxic or fear reaction is actually an allergic one,* so that the patient may be treated for the more serious condition.

Honeybees are the only one of the stinging insects whose barbed stingers remain in the human skin after the sting. A bee can only sting a patient once, for he cannot remove his stinger. Victims or sensitized persons should be instructed on the importance of removing the stinger immediately when stung by a bee. The method of removal is very important and may mean the difference between death and survival. The patient must never grasp the stinger between the thumb and forefinger or with forceps, because this method may pump more venom (antigen) from the venom sac of the stinger into the circulation and may cause a fatality. The correct removal method is to scrape or scoop the stinger out (as with a thumbnail).

The physician may be able to treat the victim better if the stinging insect is correctly identified. The nests and habitat of the insect may give a clue as to its identity. Honeybees nest in hives supplied by man, or in old dead trees, or other comparable hollow spaces. Wasps build honeycomb-type or mud nests under the eaves of houses or other areas protected from weather. Hornets build round or pear-shaped hives high in trees or bushes. Yellow jackets build their nests in the ground under logs or rocks.

Because *many victims become confused* and are unable to identify the insect that has stung them correctly, most allergists or physicians treat the patients with an extract made by mixing equal parts of materials from bees, wasps, hornets and yellow jackets.

Emergency treatment of the insect-sting-sensitive individual who has been stung by a bee, wasp, hornet involves the use of *epinephrine as quickly as possible.* The allergic person must therefore be given an *emergency treatment kit* and must receive *instruction in its use.* The kit should contain a loaded sterile syringe of epinephrine and a tourniquet. This kit should be carried by the allergic person at all times during the insect season. *The epinephrine should be used immediately after a sting and medical care should then be sought at once.* If the victim is being desensitized by a physician, then the emergency kit should be used only if some general bodily reactions occur. Tablets of *antihistamine and ephedrine,* which are contained in the emergency kit, should be swallowed by the allergic victim in addition to the other treatment.

For victims who cannot inject the syringe of epinephrine, a *vaporizer of epinephrine* may be substituted. The vaporized epinephrine is inhaled through the nose or mouth into the lungs, where the materials are rapidly absorbed.

A tourniquet may be used when the sting is on an arm or leg. Cold compresses (ice) may be helpful for local comfort. *The tourniquet may serve a double purpose:* first, absorption of the venom may be slowed down, and second, if the victim develops shock the tourniquet may keep the vein distended so that life-saving fluids may be injected intravenously by the physician.

Oxygen and a respirator may be needed if the patient does not improve. A tracheotomy (surgical opening of a breathing passage in the throat) may be necessary if obstruction of breathing occurs.

The best treatment is avoidance. The beekeeper should stop working around beehives if he has developed an allergy to bee sting. Flowers, flowering trees, and shrubs should be avoided. Bees are more likely to sting on bright, warm days, particularly following a rain that has washed nectar from the flowers. Insects are attracted to gaily-colored, dark, and rough fabrics, and not so much to white clothing with a hard finish. Bees are attracted to certain odors such as colognes, perfumes, suntan lotion, and powders. Allergic persons should not walk outdoors barefooted, since bees are attracted to clover. In fact, the amount of skin exposed should be reduced by avoiding bareheadedness, shortsleeved shirts, shorts, and bare feet. Patients should remain calm at the approach of bees and should not flail at them. Homes should have adequate screens, and garbage areas should be kept clean, so that stinging insects will not be attracted. Careful inspection of the house and its surroundings should be done at regular intervals to eradicate nests while they are still small.

In sensitive persons *desensitization treatment should be continued indefinitely*, rather than halted after two or three years. The American Academy of Allergy recommends strongly that treatment be continued indefinitely because victims have died after discontinuing treatment.

7
head injuries

Head injury represents one of the most serious consequences of an accident. Multiple, long-term effects or death may follow such an injury, but careful, systematic observations by the first aider and appropriate actions may supply the physician with information needed for rapid assessment of the patient's immediate and future status and facilitate planning for medical and surgical care.

head injuries

Buchstein, Harold F. "Head Injuries," The Journal-Lancet, 80: 375-77, August 1960.

A Clinical Assistant Professor of Neurosurgery at the University of Minnesota reports that *the motor vehicle is probably responsible for more head injuries* than any other single agent.

When a patient progressively regains consciousness following a head injury and when his respiration, blood pressure and other vital signs are only temporarily upset, it is apparent that his injury is mild or moderate. Such *an individual almost inevitably recovers.* However, he should be observed to detect any reversal in his recovery.

The severely injured patient, on the other hand, remains more or less deeply unconscious and, at times, restless for a prolonged period. There frequently is external evidence of trauma about the head accompanied by bleeding from the nose, mouth and ears. The patient may have rapid, shallow and noisy respirations, a high pulse rate, and fluctuating blood pressure. His temperature tends to rise, and he frequently exhibits neurologic abnormalities.

Shock, if present, must be combated immediately. Any serious associated injuries, particularly fractures of the spine, chest wounds, and abdominal injuries, should be treated.

The most important single consideration in the nonsurgical care of patients with head injuries is the provision of an adequate oxygen supply. The respiratory exchange of the patient with a head injury is frequently hampered by the rapid, shallow character of his breathing, and by the accumulation of fluids in the throat and larynx. There is also a tendency for the jaw and tongue to fall backward, producing mechanical obstruction. The patient should be placed on his side with his face turned toward the bed, allowing the jaw and tongue to fall forward and permitting secretions to run out of the mouth. If there is any serious degree of respiratory difficulty, a tracheotomy (by the physician or surgeon only) should be carried out immediately. This measure probably saves more lives among this group of patients than any other single maneuver. Oxygen should be administered to the patient, preferably through a tube inserted through the nose into the throat or through the tracheotomy tube (by the physician or surgeon only) if one is in place.

A rising temperature is a characteristic result of virtually every serious brain injury. If this progresses to extreme levels, it is in itself fatal. The high temperature is *neurogenic in origin* and is not necessarily evidence of infection. If the temperature rises above 103°F., it must be actively reduced. *Deliberate lowering of the temperature* to the lower 90° or upper 80° range (by means of a hypothermic blanket) *may be lifesaving.* Maintaining a state of lowered temperature for several days will help much of the swelling of the brain to recede.

There is only one real surgical emergency presented by the patient with a head injury. This is *the development of an expanding intracranial clot.* The classical example is the patient who suffers a blow to the head which produces *transient unconsciousness. He then recovers* and seems uninjured. After this so-called lucid interval, *headache, progressive coma, and partial paralysis develop. One pupil becomes dilated.* The patient's *blood pressure rises while his respiratory and pulse rates fall. Surgical removal of the clot produces a dramatic cure* if carried out before irreparable damage is done. Unfortunately, the symptoms of a blood clot in the brain are not always so clear-cut.

The patient who remains unconscious or whose coma appears to be deepening and who fails to improve *may be regarded as a candidate for surgery.* Surgery, however, can only be helpful if a space-occupying lesion of some sort is found and evacuated; that is, a blood clot or fluid accumulation of sufficient volume to compress the brain. If the patient's principal problem is injury to the brain substance itself, surgery will not benefit him.

Surgery may also be performed in other cases, such as for a depressed skull fracture. Such surgery is generally not of an emergency nature. In many of these patients, the associated brain injury is relatively mild and the patient is in no danger.

Injuries to the head differ from all other types of injuries in that they are directed toward that part of the body which, in effect, contains the patient's self and personality. The person who has received a head injury, even a minor one, may be struck by the conclusion that "I might have been killed." This is very frightening to the patient and may have far-reaching consequences in the development of symptoms arising after a head injury.

The patient should be reassured regarding the mild or minor character of his injuries *if, in the physician's opinion, this is the case.* Early ambulation is desirable. The patient should be allowed to be up just as soon as his subjective symptoms of headache, dizziness, and tendency to fatigue permit. The administration of a tranquilizing drug for a period of time may be of considerable benefit.

examination of head injuries

Oldberg, Eric. "Head Injuries," Chicago Medicine, 66: 55-56, (No. 2), January 26, 1963.

The head of the Department of Neurology of the University of Illinois College of Medicine in Chicago says that in case of head injury, *the patient's general condition and the possibility of injuries elsewhere should be explored. In the order of importance, an examination should consist of these steps:*

(1) Make an evaluation of *the patient's state of consciousness.* More

than any other one thing, the state of consciousness, the time of its appearance, and its duration is the clue to the severity of the injury.

(2) Observe whether or not the patient moves all extremities.

(3) Examine the pupils of the eyes. If the pupils are equal and the patient is conscious or semi-conscious on admission, and, if the next few hours bring a deepening of stupor and one pupil becomes markedly larger than the other, this is the best single sign indicating a blood clot, which is a surgical emergency. On the other hand, if the pupils are unequal on admission, the patient is in profound coma, and there are other pathological findings (such as paralysis or positive toe signs), then the inequality of the pupils is not so significant, except to indicate the severity of the brain damage. This is not a surgical indication. The physician will perform certain neurological tests.

(4) Toe signs are important to determine immediately, because pathological toe signs indicate definite cerebral damage.

(5) Note any leakage of blood and/or cerebrospinal fluid from the nose or ears. If fluid leakage is present, antibiotics should be started by the physician.

When this brief evaluation has been done, *the site of the blow to the head should be examined to determine whether the wound is open or closed,* whether there is compounding of the bone fracture, whether lacerated brain is extruding, and whether or not there is a depression, though the latter is almost always of minor importance from the immediate standpoint.

The patient's blood pressure, respiration, pulse rate and quality, and temperature should all be carefully recorded and watched for indications of change. If the patient is in shock, the usual measures to combat shock are in order. The less handling and moving of the patient the better. Immediate x-rays of severe, acute head injuries are rarely in order.

severe head injuries

White, Robert J., Maurice S. Albin, David Yashon and J. George Dakters. "Programmed Management of Severe Closed Head Injuries," Journal of Trauma, 8L 203-211, (No. 2), March 1968.

Four surgeons of Case-Western Reserve University School of Medicine in Cleveland, Ohio report that *persons with severe head injuries have a better chance of survival if there is an immediate diagnosis, early treatment and use of newer methods of medical management.* These surgeons base their judgment upon their experience with *52 patients* with severe closed (no open fractures) head injuries, *of which 50 survived.*

For best results there must be an immediate classification of severe head injuries into a surgical or medical need category. Obviously, it is not a function of the layman or first aider to make such a diagnosis, yet observations made at the scene of the injury may be of great value to the surgical team.

The surgeons base the *immediate diagnosis upon three sets of observations as follows: 1) a "mini"-neurological examination, 2) an estimate of the respiratory status, and 3) a medical examination.*

The mini-neurological examination concentrates on the level of consciousness and on whether or not there are critical changes taking place. The cranial nerves are examined with *specific attention to the third and seventh nerves.* The third nerve involves innervation of the pupil and the seventh nerve involves the strength of the facial muscles. Thus, *practical observations* of the pupils of the eyes and evidence of weakness of muscles of the face are helpful. First, it should be noted *whether or not the pupils differ in size and which side of the body is related to the smaller or larger pupil.* If possible *the reaction of the pupils to light should be noted* (normally, of course, the pupil gets smaller when confronted with increased light). *Mobility should also be noted:* does the pupil constrict or expand with facility, or is it fixed and immobile? Other parts of the mini-neurological examination will be conducted by the physicians, but the foregoing observations can certainly be made by helpers at the scene of the injury.

The respiratory examination involves studies of blood gases, chest films and the vital signs. For the first aider it is imperative that *observations be made of any blocking of the airway from blood, mucus, or food particles, for these obstructions must be rapidly removed.* The *nail beds* of the fingers and toes should be examined for bluish discoloration (cyanosis) which reflects concentration of reduced hemoglobin in the blood. *The type of breathing* that the patient is exhibiting should be noted also. Any variation from normal should be carefully studied and described to the physicians.

The medical examination is especially concerned with the status of the heart, condition of the lungs, and evidence of abdominal injury and suspected fracture sites. This examination is largely beyond the resource of the first-aider.

late complications in head injuries

Evans, Joseph P. "Recognition and Management of Late Complications of Head Injuries," Arizona Medicine, 25: 216-225, (No. 2), February 1968.

A professor of Neurological Surgery of the University of Chicago observes that the "late complications" of head injury depend on what happens to the head in any one of five major parts: 1) the scalp; 2) the skull; 3) the meninges (the three membranes that envelop the brain and spinal cord; 4) the brain or 5) the "psyche."

Organic or physical *damage that results from head injuries, can be classified into four major categories:* 1) scalp injuries; 2) skull fractures; 3) meningeal hemorrhage, and 4) brain injury. In addition there may be major and profound psychological implications of head injuries.

Scalp injuries are often presumed to be trivial. It should always be remembered that scalp injuries have grave *potential* significance. When hair bearing portions of the scalp is involved in the injury a wide shave of the affected area is imperative. The distribution of blood vessels of the scalp must be carefully considered when there is a head injury. It is possible that a scale infection may spread, when it is neglected, into inflammation, abscess and through penetrating veins (through the skull) into the cavity between the brain and the skull so that meningitis (inflammation of the meninges, or linings of the brain) may follow and finally, germs may spread into the actual substance of the brain itself. In one case history where the infection of a scalp injury was neglected, subsequent complications made necessary the draining of a brain abscess, an operation on the skull, the insertion of a metal plate, psychotherapy, amputation of the frontal lobe of the brain and a final total (by the age of 22 years) of 14 separate operations.

Persistent scalp tenderness after an injury is apt to reflect the trapping of nerve elements in scar tissue. Often the injection of a local anaesthetic for two or three times may bring relief.

Skull fractures of a late complication nature consist of the unrecognized depression of the skull, the onset of epilepsy, and secondary bone infections. Unrecognized depressions of the skull are rare today because of the use of x-rays in the diagnosis of head injury complications. However, when x-rays are not used for diagnostic purposes, then the depression fracture of the skull may be overlooked. *A major complication in an unrecognized depression fracture of the skull is the development of epilepsy,* which may occur in as many as 40 per cent of the cases, where there is not a proper diagnosis and treatment. Persistent headaches and dizziness after head injuries may obscure the presence of a depression fracture. Compressing depressions of the skull may disturb brain circulation and lead to later seizures.

brain damage from deceleration of the automobile

Campbell, Horace E. "Controlled Passenger Deceleration in the Automobile," Nebraska State Medical Journal, 42: 155-58 (No. 4), April 1957.

Horace E. Campbell, M.D., Chairman of the Automotive Safety Committee of the Colorado State Medical Society, observes that in automobile accidents protection of the passenger is largely a matter of preventing head injuries.

From known facts regarding the human skull it can be stated that if it is dropped upon a smooth, hard, unyielding surface from any height above five feet, a fracture is almost inevitable. Brain damage is even more likely to occur, and it is postulated that a fall from only 40 inches above a hard, unyielding surface is the upper limit of toleration. If the contacting surface is not smooth, a fall of only a foot or more, equivalent to a speed of 11 miles an hour, will result in a depressed fracture of the skull.

Thus it becomes clear who so many people are killed and injured in motor cars. There are thousands of instances where, for one reason or another, the car stops suddenly or changes direction markedly. The people keep on going at the original speed and in the original direction and come to grief upon the hard, unyielding surface of the car's interior or upon curbs, trees, fences or other similar obstacles outside the car.

Although the crash helmet has been proposed as a preventive measure for head injuries, Dr. Campbell believes that it is not a very practical solution to the problem. *It is much more practical to seek to prevent the head from striking anything.* This can be achieved by holding the motorist in his seat by means of a seat belt. The swinging forward of the head can be obviated by the wearing of a shoulder strap in addition to the seat belt. On long trips, belts and shoulder straps may be worth while just for driving comfort, quite apart from any role in injury prevention.

The instrument panel should also be so constructed and padded that it can receive the head and bring it to a stop without injury. A beginning in automobile construction has been made in this regard, but the padding is still inadequate. It is possible that the instrument panel should be abandoned on the right two-thirds of the car. It is not an essential item, as the needed instruments of the dashboard have been collected directly in front of the driver. It is Dr. Campbell's conviction that the area on the right side of the front seat should be kept as completely unoccupied space into which passengers in the front seat can swing without hitting anything at all. *It is quite possible that the automobile should be redesigned as a whole, with safety as the prime requisite.*

In present automobiles the seat belt will keep one in the car. This alone doubles the chances of survival. It also reduces the severity of head injury although it may not always prevent head injury. In a study done at Cornell of 1,039 survivors of light plane crashes, 39 of whom had forgotten to fasten their belts, head injury was present in approximately 33 per cent of the 1,000 belted survivors, and in approximately 85 per cent of the nonbelted survivors. Dangerous head injury was present in 15 per cent of the belted survivors and in 41 per cent of the 39 who had not fastened their belts.

Only nine of the 1,000 belted survivors had severe injuries due to the belt and this in spite of the fact that 221 persons actually broke their belts in the crash. *Dr. Campbell believes that safety belts would prevent 80 to 90 per cent of the current motor car fatalities.*

brain damage from head injuries

Albert S. Crawford, "Craniocerebral Injuries," Journal of the Maine Medical Association, 47: 196-97 (No. 7), July 1956.

Albert S. Crawford, M.D., Neurological Surgeon from the Veterans Administration Center at Togus, Maine, observes that *the degree and duration of unconsciousness is one of the most reliable indices of the extent of brain damage.* "Concussion" is the term applied to the least degree of damage. In concussion the duration of unconsciousness varies from a few seconds to about three hours. Patients do not die from concussion, because the brain changes are not irreversible. However, death can result from hemorrhage which develops as a later complication. "Contusion" and "laceration" are the terms applied to the more severe degrees of brain damage.

Contrary to popular conception, the fracture of the skull in itself is not the most important index of severity of the injury. It is rather the type and degree of brain damage which is significant.

The average experience in a large series of head injuries shows that about 10 per cent die in spite of the best treatment; about 70 per cent recover with an average adequate amount of treatment; and the remaining 20 per cent constitute the group which are real emergency problems. These are the cases where more or less reversible damage has occurred and where hemorrhage has supervened. In these cases survival may depend upon expert care.

Some criteria of severe brain damage are prolonged or deepening unconsciousness; progressive worsening of such vital signs as pulse, respiration, temperature, and blood pressure; continuing absence of deep tendon reflexes; fixed or dilating pupils; incontinence; and signs of increased pressure in the brain.

Cerebral hemorrhage is one of the most dreaded and dangerous of complications. Of these, the one which is more dramatic is the extradural type of brain hemorrhage which results from tearing of the middle meningeal artery. A low fracture on the side of the head is the one most likely to impair this artery. The patient normally regains his consciousness promptly and seems not to be too seriously injured. This is called the "lucid interval." During the next three to eight hours a blood clot develops, which, being outside the dura (lining of the brain) is slower in giving the telltale signs of impending danger. Pressure on the third nerve of the same side produces first constriction and, in an hour or two, progressive dilation of the pupil. Then there are slow progressive loss of consciousness, weakness of the opposite face and arm, and other neurological signs as the patient gradually subsides into deep coma. If the diagnosis can be made before the danger signs of dilated pupils, coma, and other vital abnormalities develop, and the clot is removed promptly by surgery, there is hope for a good outcome.

concussion in children

Dillon, Harold and Robert L. Leopold. "Children and the Post-Concussion Syndrome," Journal of the American Medical Association. 175: 110-16 (No. 2), January 14, 1961.

Two Philadelphia physicians engaged in the practice of neurology and psychiatry reviewed 60 medical reports published since 1954 and found very little concerning head injuries to children, although a few investigators pointed out that different reactions occur to head injuries in adults and in children.

The two physicians then studied 50 children (35 boys and 15 girls) during 1959 and 1960, all of whom had been in accidents in which a medical diagnosis of concussion (and in 20 cases certain other associated injuries) had been made.

There are three major reactions to concussion of the brain in *adults,* as follows: 1) headache; 2) dizziness, and 3) irritability.

This study reveals that children rarely show the same symptoms as adults following head injuries that result in concussion and loss of consciousness.

In 13 of the children no headache whatsoever occurred. In the remaining 37 children only mild headaches of short duration were recorded. In not one case was a severe, persistent headache of the adult type observed or recorded.

Symptoms of dizziness occurred in only 9 of the 50 children, even when there was associated damage to the ear.

Ocular (visual) symptoms occurred in 14 children, varying from double vision, burning, pain and blurring of vision to puffiness.

Physical symptoms of concussions in children were found to be far less important and of lesser severity and duration in children.

In 47 of the 50 children (over 90 per cent) there were marked psychological changes (behavior changes), such as: tension (28); restlessness (26); nightmares and frightening dreams (14); loss of bladder control (13); withdrawal and regression (8); "queer" behavior (7); aggressive behavior (6); fear of autos (5); difficulty in management (4); fear of being alone (4); sluggishness (3); antisocial acts as breaking things, playing with fire (2); temper tantrums (1). Eight students showed moderate to serious deterioration in school work.

Eight of the 50 children developed convulsive seizures. Of 25 children on whom electroencephalograms were taken 11 were moderately or maximally abnormal.

results of severe head injuries in childhood

Hjern, B. and Ingvar Nylander. "Late Prognosis of Severe Head Injuries in Children," Archives of Disease in Childhood, 37: 113-16, (No. 192), April 1962.

Two physicians from Stockholm, Sweden, report *a study of 22 children* between the ages of one and fourteen years of age who were treated in that city for *severe head injuries* during a ten year period. These severely injured children had been followed for a period of six months to nine and a half years after the injury.

In these severe head injuries the children remained unconscious for from one to 50 days.

It was found that *with nine children out of the total of 22 there were no serious neurological or psychiatric results*. Three of the children have been found to have a completely normal status and six others have had slight symptoms which could be due to causes other than the head injury. Of the remaining *13 children the results have been more serious*. One boy now has a pronounced case of *cerebral palsy* and *intellectual retardation*. Another boy has pronounced difficulties in school and with companions due to *personality alteration* and intellectual retardation. A girl has slight cerebral palsy, but her personality alteration has been so severe that she cannot be cared for at home at times. One girl has partially *diminished hearing, psychomotor epilepsy* and other changes. One boy has lost the feeling of *sensation* in half of his face and is *totally deaf* in one ear. Another boy has a *facial* paralysis and moderate *loss of muscular strength* in the extremities. Seven children have slight symptoms including *slight paralysis of hands or feet,* impaired hearing and *speech disturbance.* Certain *psychological changes* have also occurred in this group.

At the time of discharge following initial treatment some of the children showed grave psychiatric symptoms, but at the time of the follow-up investigation they were symptom-free. According to information which appeared to be reliable *improvements came as much as three years after the head injury.*

emergency care of facial injuries

Eade, Gilbert G. "Emergency Care of Facial Injuries," Northwest Medicine, 68: 729-737, (No. 8), August 1969.

A Seattle, Washington physician in a presentation at the annual meeting of the Seattle Surgical Society, recited his own *medical and surgical experience in the treatment of 1,000 cases of fractures of the face.*

Out of this rich experience he found that about *two-thirds of all facial fractures occurred in automobile accidents.* About 4 per cent of the 1,000 cases had massive injuries to the face, such as crushing, smashing injuries much like what happens to the shell of a hard-boiled egg if it is stepped on.

One thing that Dr. Eade emphasizes is that patients are not injured teeth or injured faces—they are injured *people. Of the 42 patients (4 per cent) with massive injuries to the face,* all had an associated head injury. Of this group 38 per cent died, or 16 of the 42 badly damaged patients.

In a massive face injury if the patient is restless he has difficulty in breathing.

There are three major problems in the treatment of persons with facial injuries: 1) breathing; 2) bleeding and 3) a missed diagnosis by the physician, according to Dr. Eade.

Airway, or breathing problems, take precedence over all other consideration in the person with a facial injury. Food, vomitus, mucus, blood clots, bleeding, broken dentures or tooth fragments can all interfere with breathing. An immediate cause of death should never be an inability to breathe. The insertion of a tube through the mouth by the physician or first aider is fast, easy, and not harmful. It may save a life.

Bleeding is next in importance after breathing. Rapid and significant blood loss can occur, although it is not common in facial injuries. Bleeding must be controlled.

A missed diagnosis is next in importance. An Indian girl with massive face injury, skull fracture, fractured pelvis and a dislocated hip, died after treatment for these injuries, from a ruptured spleen. However, in serious, multiple injuries the most life-threatening problems must be treated first. Often missed in diagnosis is a serious neck injury. Every patient with a smashed face injury should be considered as having a serious neck injury until it is proven otherwise. *Transportation carts are needed from which x-rays can be taken without moving the patient.*

injuries to the face

Taddeo, Ronald J., Charles E. Horton, Jerome E. Adamson, Richard Mladick and Cephas N. Christian. "The Management of Facial Bone Fractures," Ohio State Medical Journal, 65: 899-904, (No. 9), September 1969.

Five physicians of the Norfolk General Hospital in Virginia observe that *as automobiles are increasing, so is the incidence of fractures of the bones of the face.* Automobile accidents now constitute the greatest single cause of such injuries. Even seat belts have increased facial injuries because the face is often thrown against the dashboard in automobile accidents.

Even a severely fractured face may appear to be relatively undamaged. The face should be carefully examined in respect to its symmetrical appearance, or lack of it. Bony irregularities may be apparent at early examination, whereas later, severe swelling all over the face may make it difficult to detect injury that could be recognized at first.

Emergency treatment must be first directed at the maintenance of breathing. Swelling that may close up the air passages can occur in face and neck injuries. Also, bony obstruction, blood clots, hemorrhage, and foreign bodies such as loose teeth, dentures, glass and debris must be looked for in all cases of injury to the face, especially if the victim has a reduced level of consciousness, for breathing may be obstructed.

For active bleeding the application of temporary compression packs may be life saving.

If what looks like clear mucus is dripping from the nose, it is likely to be cerebrospinal fluid and probably indicates a fracture through a skull bone (cribriform plate). If a patient sees double or suffers from numbness over the cheek or upper lip there is the possibility of a blowout fracture of the orbit (broken bone in the eye socket).

In facial injuries an examination of the teeth is very important. The presence of teeth is a basic foundation for the repair of a severely fractured face. If the teeth are sound the jaw can be used for stabilization of other broken bones of the face. Even broken dentures (false teeth) should not be discarded because they may be used in later stabilization of other broken bones.

X-rays should always be taken. However, in injuries to the nose, the clinical examination and general medical impressions are more important than x-rays, for the latter may not be diagnostic. Nasal bones can be treated for up to two weeks, so they should be treated before swelling occurs or after it subsides.

broken nose in childhood

Capo, Oscar A. "Nasal Fractures in Children," Ohio State Medical Journal, 65: 905, (No. 9), September 1969.

An ear, nose and throat specialist of the University of Cincinnati College of Medicine reports that *an unrecognized and untreated fracture of the nose in children is of the greatest importance.* If a broken nose in a child is not suspected, and therefore not treated, the normal growth and development of the structures of the face may be impaired seriously. *The damage may not be apparent* until adolescent development results in gross nasal deformity.

X-rays may be helpful, but often they show no damage in the usual views. A description of how the injury occurred is helpful, but *most important of all is the careful examination of the injured child.*

Fracture and displacement of the cartilage of the nose may occur independently of bone injury. This kind of injury occurs only in children, but it is very common. Fracture of either the cartilage or the bone that goes unrecognized and untreated becomes apparent in adult life by both internal and external deformities of the nose.

Any child who has nosebleed following an injury to the nose can be assumed to have a fracture. If there is a rupture of the nasal mucosa (internal lining of the nose) or if a blood tumor (hematoma) can be seen, these signs are highly suggestive of fractures. Any blood tumors (hematomas) must be treated soon because infection may develop and be followed by destruction of cartilage with later deformities.

The cartilage and bone of the nasal structures in children may be broken, displaced without fracture, or may be telescoped in such a way as to cause overlapping and later abnormal development.

Nasal fractures in children are often overlooked and go untreated because it is believed they are insignificant. Such is not the case. If a fracture is suspected the physician is justified in placing the child under anesthesia so that he can elevate and manipulate the nasal tissues to see if there are fractures or dislocations. Corrections can be made by placing the tissues back in proper position and supporting them with packs and splints if necessary.

loss of hearing from head injury

Does, I.E.A. and T. Bottema. "Postraumatic Conductive Hearing Loss," Archives of Otolaryngology, 82: 331-339, (No. 4), October 1965.

Two physicians of the University of Utrecht in the Netherlands report *a study of 15 persons who had impaired hearing as a result of injury to the head.* The increasing frequency of traffic accidents, in which head injuries may occur, is cited as a matter of importance by the Dutch physicians in respect to the loss of hearing.

So far as hearing is concerned, *an injury in which the temple is fractured is most important,* because fractures of the petrosal bone (side of the head above the cheek bone) are apt to damage the middle ear, while the deeper or inner ear parts are left intact. A fracture in the side of the head (temporal area) may cause a rupture of the eardrum and facial nerve paralysis or a hemorrhage into the area of the eardrum.

broken eardrums in children

Spector, Martin. "Tympanic Membrane Perforations in Children," Clinical Pediatrics, 3: 25-27 (No. 1), January 1964.

An ear specialist from the Temple Medical School of Philadelphia observes that *broken eardrums are caused by injury or infection.* In children the *chief cause is an infection* of the middle ear (otitis media). Less often, an injury to the ear from a direct blow, blast, concussion or head injury may cause the rupture. External ear infections rarely cause a perforation. Occasionally a small tumor of cholesterol and fat may be the source of a perforation.

The majority of broken eardrums tend to heal *spontaneously,* but chronic perforations lead to trouble in two ways: repeated infections of the ear and loss of hearing.

Surgical correction of a ruptured eardrum should be sought if the perforation has persisted for three to six months *after all* infection has been cleared from the ear, or if there has been a loss of hearing. If infections occur because water gets into the middle ear surgery should be done also.

Surgery should not be done if an infection cannot be cleared up, if there is a blocked Eustachian tube, or if a tumor cannot be completely removed. If an infection or tumor is buried under the surgeon's graft the troubles of the patient are aggravated rather than alleviated. If the Eustachian tube is blocked then closure of the broken eardrum results in persistent, serious infection of the middle ear (otitis media).

Vein tissue is a satisfactory grafting material at all ages for the closing of the space of a ruptured eardrum, but Fascia is an even more useful repair tissue and can be secured in quantities great enough to close even a massive perforation.

The invention of the operating binocular microscope (which provides binocular vision, magnifies 6 to 16 times, and gives ample light) has been a boon to all otologists (ear specialists). Other advances have also helped.

After the eardrum has been grafted the patient may leave the hospital in a day or two, but should be seen weekly since some discharge or secretion may need to be removed by the doctor. The graft surface is not cleared for 3 weeks because of the hazard of removal. There is relatively little discomfort in this kind of surgery and the graft is successful in about 90 per cent of the cases.

8
psychiatric emergencies

Many of the signs and symptoms of psychiatric emergencies are unrecognized by the layman, and even the signs of an impending suicide may go unheeded. The psychiatric emergency is as important to the person rendering first aid as any other condition that may threaten life or health.

The simple techniques of emergency psychotherapy should be a part of the knowledge of all well-trained first aiders, and the signs and symptoms that call for such procedures should be well understood.

psychiatric symptoms of children

Shechtman, Audrey. "Psychiatric Symptoms Observed in Normal and Disturbed Children," Journal of Clinical Psychology, 26: 38-41, (No. 1), January 1970.

A researcher from DePaul University in Illinois reports on a *comparison of behavioral symptoms* found in a group of 62 children (25 boys and 37 girls) admitted to a mental health clinic as compared to behaviors observed in a matched group of "normal" children. Ages ranged from six through 13.

Criteria for selection as "normal" were no history of problem behavior in the classroom or community, no history of psychiatric contact, and functioning close to a level commensurate with intellectual ability. The normal children were matched with the clinic children with regard to age, sex, level of education, and occupation of the supporting parent.

Ashenbach's 91 item checklist of behaviors frequently associated with psychiatric disorders in children was used.

The clinic children showed a greater number of symptoms than the controls, but overlap between the two groups was marked. However,

21 differentiating symptoms were found in the disturbed children, such as: "bizarre behavior, can't concentrate, cruelty, daydreaming, depression, disobedience, excessive talking, fighting, loudness, lying, masochism (suicidal), negativism, phobias, poor schoolwork, restlessness, running away, stealing, temper tantrums, tics, vomiting, and worrying." In addition, clinic children often had previous problems, or parents with problems, and they functioned at a lower level in school.

Apparently, *while many child behaviors have a high nuisance value* for adults, only a few (and those are relatively severe) distinguish the mentally disturbed child from the one who is functioning more adequately. The remainder of the behavioral symptoms are evidenced by most normal children, although with lesser frequency, intensity, and at more appropriate age levels. *Presence of the symptoms themselves, then, is not* necessarily indicative of a need for professional psychiatric help.

A wide range of symptoms frequently associated with psychiatric disorders is found in relatively normal children, but only a few indicate the child with severe problems.

emergency psychotherapy

Bellak, Leopold. *"The Role and Nature of Emergency Psychotherapy," American Journal of Public Health, 58: 344-347 (No. 2), February 1968.*

A visiting clinical professor of psychiatry at New York University observes that it is surprising that emergency psychiatric care should be a relatively new development. The importance of emotional disorders has not been fully acknowledged.

Even today, the emergency psychiatric clinic of the walk-in type is still a rarity, according to Dr. Bellak.

The purpose of emergency psychotherapy is to alleviate pain, make functioning possible, and to save life. Emergency psychotherapy is intended not only to protect the individual against the loss of the patient through suicide, but also the protection of other lives in crippling emotional situations.

An essential element in emergency psychotherapy is the discovery of acute cases. The family doctor, policemen, lawyers, teachers, the clergy, hospital administrators and others are sources for detection.

Emotional care on an emergency basis may be able to prevent an acute disorder from becoming a chronic one. The financial aspects of the latter public health problem alone must be figured in the billions. Half of all the hospital beds in the United States are still taken by psychiatric patients. Even if there is not hospitalization, chronic emotional illness accounts for a staggering amount of decreased functioning in society.

Emergency psychiatric care must be available twenty-four hours a day.

The nature of emergency psychotherapy must depend upon the particular case. An exploration of fantasies, fears and guilt may be necessary. Sedation may be advisable. Intellectual clarification of a situation may be needed. A few group-psychotherapy sessions may be needed for groups that have gone through emotionally disturbing experiences. Joint interviews with husband and wife may be appropriate. Tranquilizers may be needed to control acute excitement. Emergency psychotherapy must be flexible, but there must be a systematic foundation.

brief psychotherapy*

Castelnuovo-Tedesco, Pietro. "Brief Psychotherapy: Current Status," California Medicine, 107: 263-269, (No. 3), September 1967.

The Chief of the Department of Psychiatry of the Harbor General Hospital in Torrance, California, observes that brief psychotherapy is intended to relieve the patient's suffering, and, in particular, his most pressing and disabling symptoms, as promptly and expeditiously as possible. Value is placed on brevity and economy of treatment.

Deliberate attention is paid to the patient's major conflicts and to the

*Oliver E. Byrd, *Medical Readings on Drug Abuse*, 1970, Addison-Wesley, Reading, Mass.

key relationships involved in the patient's current upset. The emphasis is on taking care of first things first.

A wide variety of techniques is available to achieve the goals of treatment, such as the following:

(1) The rapid establishment of *a warm, positive relationship*, between the patient and the psychiatrist.

(2) Ventilation (the open discussion of grievances) and emotional catharsis *(purging the mind of repressed material)*.

(3) Reassurance and suggestion.

(4) Counseling, advice, exhortation, and environmental manipulation.

(5) Explanation and educational remarks.

(6) Drug-giving

(7) Interpretative maneuvers, such as *clarification of feelings, thoughts, and attitudes*, confrontations (bringing two patients together for diagnostic purposes), and so on.

(8) Desensitization by counter-conditioning techniques, especially for phobias and other focal anxiety responses.

Brief psychotherapy has much to offer, yet *it is not suitable for all patients or all conditions,* and there are some situations where it is quite unsuitable. It is best limited to persons of reasonably mature personality and adequate motivation, where emotional disturbances are not chronic, or less than of extreme intensity. It is best for *neurotic* patients, rather than those who are grossly incapacitated. Those persons who suffer from anxiety, moderate depression, or minor hysterical conversions frequently respond remarkably well. Psychotic patients, or those with massive character disorders; alcoholics, drug addicts, severely unstable persons, or those with disabling "psychosomatic illnesses" such as ulcerative colitis and so on do not respond well. *Special care must be taken with suicidal risks, as brief treatment may not offer enough protection.* Poorest results are obtained with the sickest people.

emotional disorders and traffic accidents

Selzer, Melvin L., Joseph E. Rogers and Sue Kern. "Fatal Accidents: The Role of Psychopathology, Social Stress, and Acute Disturbance," American Journal of Psychiatry, 124: 1028-1036 (No. 8), February 1968.

Two physicians and a social worker of the Department of Psychiatry of the University of Michigan Medical Center at Ann Arbor report a study of *96 automobile drivers who were responsible for fatal accidents* over a period of three years. A control group of 96 other drivers was used for comparative purposes.

In this investigation *three sources of emotional disturbance* were revealed: 1) chronic emotional disorders; 2) some form of social stress and 3) an acutely disturbing experience that occurred before the accident.

Alcohol-addicted drivers were also much more prevalent in the fatal accident driving group than in the control drivers.

In the fatal-accident group of drivers 23 per cent were found to have *paranoid ideas* as compared to 5 per cent in the other group of drivers. Twenty-one per cent of the fatality group had *tendencies toward suicide,* as compared to 8 per cent. Twenty-one per cent also had experienced clinical *depression* as compared to 8 per cent of the control group.

Social stress, such as a serious and disturbing personal conflict or a job or money crisis during 12 months before the fatal accident, was more prevalent in the fatality group. Of the latter, 32 per cent had more *personal conflicts,* 36 per cent had *vocational or financial stresses* and 20 per cent had disturbing experiences, such as *quarrels,* within 6 hours of the fatal accident.

Most of the disturbing experiences before the accident consisted of *violent quarrels with wives, girl-friends, barmaids or female drinking companions. A few physical fights had occurred with other men.*

This study reveals that *a multiplicity of emotional factors may contribute to a fatal accident.* Chronic emotional problems, acute and chronic social stress and preaccident disturbances all seem to vie for relationships to the accident. *For example,* a 22-year-old married factory worker had violent and quarrelsome relations with his wife, paranoid suspicions regarding his wife's relationships with other men. He had a violent temper and once when intoxicated savagely beat a young man. In deep remorse he took four sleeping pills in a suicide attempt. The day before the accident his wife left him with their infant daughter, he drank a half pint of bourbon and later had five double bourbons at a bar within 25 minutes. He went to another bar and drank some more. He started home at a high rate of speed and killed the driver of another car as he was turning off the highway. The relationships of paranoia, violence, suicidal impulse, a nightmare marriage, and a disturbing quarrel prior to the accident are all apparent. This man was still driving an automobile at the time of this report.

the potential suicide

Naftulin, Donald H. "The Potentially Suicidal Patient," California Medicine, III: 169-176, (No. 3), September 1969.

A physician of the Department of Psychiatry of the University of Southern California School of Medicine observes that *today suicide ranks as the tenth major cause of death* and that about 20,000 persons are known to kill themselves each year. There may be about 50,000 deaths by suicide each year, for many of them may be concealed for family reasons or may be mistaken for an accident or other cause.

Patients who come to a physician for the first time should be assessed for their capacity to deal with stress. For example, if the loss of a job, a loved one, or the patient's self-esteem has been followed by *mourning, despair, or apathy for longer than six to 12 weeks* then more attention should be paid to other factors that may reflect reactions to stress. If *anxiety, weight loss, insomnia, fatigue, social withdrawal* and other reactions have lingered long after the loss then it is significant to discover if they represent a new pattern of behavior or if they are results that always follow stressful situations for the patient. If the reactions are typical then it is important to explore in a tactful way any previous suicidal thoughts or attempts.

If a person has considered suicide in the past, then there are six clues as to the risk of suicide in the future: 1) How frequent and extensively has the person had suicidal thoughts? 2) Has he ever considered how he would commit suicide? 3) What feelings were associated with thinking about the ways in which suicide might be achieved? 4) Are the methods thought about available for carrying out the idea of suicide? 5) What feelings of suicide, if any, accompany ordinary acts of everyday life? 6) Is the potential suicide able to understand how loved ones would be affected by his death?

To communicate with a person who is contemplating suicide one must listen. The person should not be accused, but should be understood and encouraged to talk. Often the suicidal risk will have passed after about six weeks, which is the usual duration of emotional crises or reactions to loss. Thus, for six weeks one should be willing to listen, so that the patient can "ventilate" his feelings. From 15 to 20 minutes per week is usually enough if the risk of suicide is judged to be relatively low.

Progress is being made when feelings have diminished in intensity, when the patient has gotten rid of things with which he can commit suicide, such as lethal pills, when appetite and sleeping patterns have improved and when there is less brooding. Depression is not among the clinical signs of the high-risk potential suicide. The highest risk category is those who have decided that suicide is the logical solution to conflict.

attempted suicides

Dorpat, Theodore L. and John W. Boswell. "An Evaluation of Suicidal Intent in Suicide Attempts," *Comprehensive Psychiatry, 4: 117-25 (No. 2), April 1963.*

Two members of the Department of Psychiatry of the University of Washington School of Medicine in Seattle have reported on a study of 121 attempted suicides in an effort to discover the real intent of the victims. A comparison was made with 114 completed suicides.

Three different types of suicidal behavior were found in this research, as follows:

1 *The serious attempt* group was found to be depressed, to have a feeling of hopelessness and to show a lack of social interaction. Severity of intent was found to increase with age. Approximately one-third of the group was found to be psychotic. Usually the suicide act was deliberate after careful planning. The loss of loved ones and serious illness were leading factors.

2 *The confused, vacillating* group usually provided a means for their own rescue by notifying others of their intentions, by taking dosages of sleeping pills or other substances that would not kill them, or by timing their attempt at suicide in such a way that they would be rescued. Despite their confusion the members of this group appeared to be testing the affection and care of others.

3 *The suicide gesture group.* The members of this suicide group sought to make others feel guilty and ashamed. Their attempts were merely a gesture for a variety of reasons, such as seeking release from jail, trying to get into a hospital, trying to avoid the draft or to prevent divorce or separation. Over one-half of these "gesture" suicides were precipitated by a quarrel. Often the thwarted lover was found to attempt suicide to gain attention, love, or marriage. Not infrequently such an action succeeds in gaining of the objective. The members of this suicide group have no intention of dying. Their object is to manipulate others and to enforce a closer bond with the object of their action.

attempted suicides in adolescents

Senseman, Laurence A. "Attempted Suicide in Adolescents," Rhode Island Medical Journal, 51: 109-112, (No. 2), February 1968.

A physician and Medical Director of the Fuller Sanitarium of South Attleboro, Massachusetts, reports *a continuing study of 100 young people between the ages of 14 and 21* who have been admitted to the Fuller Memorial Sanitarium. Of this number *56 had threatened or attempted suicide.*

Suicide is one of the 12 leading causes of death in the United States and *ranks second as a cause of death among college students.* In the age *group 15 to 19 years suicide is the third leading cause of death.* Although death from suicide occurs about every 20 minutes in the United States, it is estimated that there are *at least five unsuccessful attempts for every successful one.*

Most children who destroy themselves, or try to do so, feel that suicide is their only way out of a difficult situation. *All suicide attempts should be taken seriously,* and should be treated promptly with medical and psychiatric care. The rate of successful suicide increases with repeated attempts. Difficulties with parents, peers, poverty, pregnancy and broken homes have a high relationship to suicides.

In this study schizophrenia, depression reaction, anxiety reaction, depression after childbirth, personality disorder, character disorder, and reactions of adolescence were associated with the suicide attempts. It should be obvious that *mental illness may* predispose to an attempted suicide. Nearly everything gets blamed for suicide: love, hate, religion, pain, boredom, fear, shame, guilt, welfare, a new job, the boss, the time of year and even the weather.

Four factors are of significance in the possibility of suicide: 1) *the thought;* 2) *the* means; 3) *the action* and 4) *the attempt.* If only the thought is present, on careful questioning the physician need not be greatly concerned, but should check on the matter later. If positive answers are given by the patient as to the means by which he may commit suicide, then the physician has some responsiblity (which he should share with a relative), because the risk of suicide is greater. There may be a world of difference between thought and action, but if the patient has taken any action in preparation for suicide, then the responsibility of the physician becomes strong. He must share his concern with the family and he should recommend psychiatric care. If there has been an actual attempt at suicide, then the likelihood of another attempt is greatly accentuated. Hospitalization is required, relatives must be consulted, and psychiatric consultation must be held.

The above approach should be helpful in evaluating the young person in respect to possible suicide. He may seek help, but he may not reveal all of his feelings. He should be questioned about his thoughts, the means he might use for suicide, whether or not he has taken any action toward suicide, and whether he has ever attempted suicide.

delinquency and accidents

Klein, David. "Some Applications of Delinquency Theory to Childhood Accidents," Pediatrics, 44: 805-810, (No. 5, Part II), November 1969.

David Klein, of the Department of Social Science at Michigan State University, observes that *delinquency and childhood accidents are both forms* or consequences *of deviant behavior* and have many similarities.

The earliest theories of delinquency sought the explanation in "organic defects" in the individual. It was also believed that the child with physical or mental handicaps was more likely to be "accident prone." Both these theories have been carefully demolished by careful demonstration that neither delinquents nor accident victims are distinguishable in terms of physical characteristics.

Other theories have implicated the child's parents, siblings, and other relatives. For instance, psychologists readily recognize parents whose authoritarian rigidity forces the children into delinquency, and the overprotective but rejecting parent whose child seems destined to become an accident victim. This type of theory, however, ignores the broader social environment. *Neither delinquents nor accident victims can be reliably distinguished through psychological measurement,* no matter how refined.

Sociological theories insist that it is the interaction of physical and psychological characteristics with the social environment that encourages or inhibits delinquency and accidents. There are many variations of such theories.

One such theory is that *every society teaches its members to value certain goals,* such as wealth, athletic prowess, academic ability, and leadership. *But society does not give all its members equal opportunity* to reach these goals. Those people who cannot attain them legitimately are likely to achieve them by deviant means, if they do not reject the goals entirely.

The child who fails to gain parental attention may injure himself in an accident, or engage in risk taking and daredevil behavior to gain peer-group status. In other words, in trying to meet our expectations, *some children use delinquent behavior; others have accidents.*

In any one area delinquency and accidents are likely to be inversely related—that is, *the neighborhood reporting a high delinquency rate is likely to report a low childhood accident rate.* The author believes that this difference does not infer that the underlying causes are different, but on the contrary furnishes excellent sociological evidence to indicate that the causes of delinquency and childhood accidents are similar.

psychiatric emergencies in children*

Mattsson, Ake, James W. Hawkins and Lynne R. Seese. "Child Psychiatric Emergencies," Archives of General Psychiatry, 17: 584-592 (No. 5), November 1967.

Three staff members of the School of Medicine and University Hospitals of Western Reserve University, Cleveland, Ohio, report on a

*Oliver E. Byrd, *Medical Readings on Drug Abuse,* 1970, Addison-Wesley, Reading, Mass.

study of 170 children admitted to the child psychiatry clinic for emergency treatment. The purpose of the study was to determine what kind of children have psychiatric emergencies and how effective treatment may be.

A child psychiatric emergency is defined by the investigators as a condition of *sufficient emotional distress in a child that it cannot be handled for even a few hours by the child himself, his family, or by others from whom help may be sought.* Although the ages of the children in this study ranged from four to approximately 18 years, *the greatest concentration* of psychiatric emergencies occurred *in the 15 to 18 year old group.* Among these patients *girls outnumbered boys in a ratio of three to one* and 50 per cent of the girls were referred to the clinic because an an attempt at suicide.

In the total group, *suicidal behavior was by far the largest single psychiatric emergency,* occurring in 75 cases. The suicidal acts of the boys were of a more serious nature and more associated with a state of depression than was the case with the girls. In the case of the latter the suicidal attempt or gesture often reflected an impulsive, rebellious, or frightening and manipulative effort to control parents or loved ones.

Three-fourths of the 170 children with psychiatric emergencies were found to have had at least one year's history of emotional disorder. In fact, psychosocial pathology had caused the parents of these children to be *known to various community agencies for years.* After emergency treatment, *one-third of all the children were admitted to a psychiatric ward for sustained treatment* and another one-third accepted more extended psychiatric treatment on an out-patient basis. In general, suicidal behavior, incipient psychosis (serious mental illness) and acute school refusal represented genuine psychiatric emergencies in the children.

The crucial events that triggered the psychiatric emergencies in this group of 170 children were as follows: 1) Arguments, fights, abuse involving conflicts between child and parents, 54 cases; 2) exacerbations of physical illness or injuries, including surgery, 25 cases; 3) school problems, 17 cases; 4) sexual conflicts involving masturbation, menstruation, and homosexual contacts, 17 cases; 5) conflict with or loss of a loved one of opposite sex, 12 cases; 6) pregnancy, 9 cases; 7) grief reactions, 8 cases; 8) intoxication, 6 cases; and 9) sexual molestation, 3 cases.

Emergency service programs call for: 1) prompt diagnosis; 2) clarification for the family of precipitating factors; 3) involvement of parents in treatment; 4) access to psychiatric inpatient treatment; 5) clinic facilities for continued treatment; 6) close cooperation with community resources; 7) flexible schedules for psychiatric workers and 8) recognition of the need for an emergency plan and service.

child abuse

Gil, David G. *"Physical Abuse of Children—Findings and Implications of a Nationwide Survey," Pediatrics, 44: 857-864, (No. 5, Part II), November 1969.*

David Gil, of the Florence Heller Graduate School for Advanced Studies in Social Welfare at Brandeis University, points out that *some children have always been subjected to a wide range of physical abuse by parents* and other caretakers.

The types of injuries range from minor bruises and cuts to burns, scaldings, fractures, internal injuries, intentional starvation, dismemberment, and severe injuries to the brain and central nervous system.

The growing awareness of child abuse led *during the 1960's* to the enactment by all states of *laws requiring medical personnel* and others *to report incidents of suspected abuse* to appropriate authorities.

During 1967, *a nationwide total of 5,993 physically abused children was legally reported.* Slightly more than half of the children were boys. Two-thirds of all the children were white, and one-third were non-white. Nearly 30 per cent of the children displayed noticeable deviations in social and behavioral functioning.

Nearly 30 per cent of the children lived in families without a father. The educational level, occupational status, and income of the parents were very low. The number of children in the families tended to be higher than the national average. Over 40 per cent of the mothers and 45 per cent of the fathers were rated deviant in social functioning.

The injuries of the children were rated "not serious" in 53 per cent of the incidents. In 37 per cent, they were rated serious without permanent damage. Five per cent were rated serious with permanent damage, and four per cent were fatal. Sixty-three per cent of the incidents arose out of disciplinary action taken by a parent.

In some cases, abuse was an expression of a severe personality disorder on the part of the attacker. Broken families and environmental strains such as those related to poverty were significantly associated with child abuse. Some children, because of unusual congenital or acquired characteristics, may occasionally be more likely to provoke abuse attacks against themselves than other more "normal" children.

Although the cases of child abuse are no doubt under reported, 5,993 reported cases per year in a nation of 200 million do not constitute a major social problem, at least in relative terms, tragic as every single incident may be. *The classical "battered child syndrome" is a relatively infrequent occurrence.*

9
drug reactions

Drug reactions range from mild to severe. Many of them can be treated successfully only by the physician, but some can be handled by the layman or the first aider effectively until psychiatric or medical care becomes available. In fact, the early observations of the first aider may be of great importance to the physician in determining the cause of the reaction and what kind of medical or psychiatric care should be rendered.

emergency care for drug reactions

Holcenberg, John S. and Lawrence M. Halpern. "Drug Therapy: II Treatment of Drug Misuse," Northwest Medicine, 69: 31-33, (No. 1), January 1970.

A physician and a pharmacologist of the University of Washington School of Medicine in Seattle discuss the treatment of various categories of drug reactions. These are some of their conclusions:

1 *Solvent inhalation.* Harmful effects of vapor sniffing differ according to the substance that is inhaled, but the greatest danger appears to be suffocation in a plastic bag. Emergency care of acute, severe intoxication requires the establishment of adequate ventilation (artificial respiration) and observation for toxic side effects.

2 *Stimulant drugs.* Overdosage with amphetamines is apt to cause disorganized behavior, inability to sleep, paranoid ideas which may lead to violent acts, hallucinations and other symptoms. Withdrawal may present a serious psychiatric problem with depression, fatigue, sleepiness and hunger for about a week. Patients must be watched for suicide attempts. Sedatives, tranquilizers, or mood elevators should be avoided, because little is known about possible drug reactions in over-dosage with amphetamines.

3 *Sedatives, hypnotics and minor tranquilizers.* These drugs may accentuate the depressant effects of each other and the latter may be further emphasized if alcohol, antihistamines, or phenothiazines are taken. These drugs are hazardous because they may alter the metabolism of other drugs as well as having their own depressant effects. Proper care calls for hospitalization in an intensive care unit that gives support to respiration, treatment of shock and the use of antibiotics to prevent pneumonia. Barbiturate overdosage, followed by removal from the drug, may lead to convulsions, which should be prevented in a hospital with declining dosages of the drug.

4 *Hallucinogenic drugs.* Bad trips are relatively low in occurrence and are best treated by a sympathetic, calm person who gives reassurance. Rarely is any drug treatment needed.

5 *Narcotics.* Nalorphine (Nalline) can be used to counter respiratory depression caused by the opiate drugs, but it has a relatively short duration of action and must be given repeatedly. Nalorphine must be used with extreme caution by the physician since it may cause an exaggerated withdrawal reaction with convulsions. Otherwise, treatment is much the same as with the sedatives (see above) with declining dosages of the drug to which the patient is addicted.

6 *Marijuana.* Infrequently, marijuana users may show stomach upsets, paranoid agitation and hysterical rigidity of several hours duration, according to the authors. Reassurance and bed rest seem adequate. The long term effects of marijuana are not known.

barbiturate overdosage[*]

Baker, A. B. "Early Treatment of the Unconscious Patient Suffering from Drug Overdosage," Medical Journal of Australia, 1: 56th Year· 497-503, (No. 10), March 8, 1969.

An Australian physician of the Royal Brisbane Hospital reports that *in Australia as many as one person in every eight may attempt suicide*

[*]Oliver E. Byrd, *Medical Readings on Drug Abuse*, 1970, Addison-Wesley, Reading, Mass.

by taking drugs. Most commonly the drug taken is a barbiturate alone or in combination with another drug. (The first death from an overdosage of a barbiturate occurred in 1905, although not in Australia.)

Over a period of 21 months all of the patients admitted to the Respiratory Unit of the hospital with a diagnosis of drug-overdose were studied by the author. During this time *553 patients were admitted in an unconscious state due to drug overdosage.* It was not possible in each case to discover which drug had been used, but where the drugs were identified, the most commonly used were the barbiturates. Often other drugs were taken in combination.

Modern medical methods to save the lives of persons suffering from an overdose of barbiturates began to be used between 1940 and 1950. Treatment emphasized the maintenance of breathing, circulation and body minerals (electrolytes) while the body was excreting the drug by natural means. After about 1960, however, more vigorous methods began to be used by the physician, based upon physiological principles. Forced excretion of urine to help remove the drug; alkalinization of the urine by drugs designed to overcome the acid condition of barbiturate poisoning; exchange transfusions of blood; the passage of the blood of the patient over charcoal for absorption of toxic drugs, and other measures began to be used. The deaths from drug overdosage fell from about 20 per cent to 1 or 2 per cent with these methods of treatment.

Today, more and more methods are being used to hasten excretion of the drug. The surgical insertion of a tube into the throat to assist breathing (tracheal intubation), the control of breathing by a mechanical ventilator, blood gas analyses and other procedures are used to help the patient recover, such as the rapid use of digitalis or some other substance if the heart begins to fail. Fluid is given by vein and falling blood pressure is watched for; efforts are also made to prevent lung infections.

Under the foregoing vigorous medical treatment *only 4 of the 553 patients died. All four were suffering from barbiturate overdosage.* Slightly under 1 per cent of the patients died from barbiturate overdosage under the treatments indicated, which were less intensive than procedures used in some hospitals.

handling of bad trips

Taylor, Robert L., John I. Maurer and Jared R. Tinklenberg. "Management of Bad Trips in an Evolving Drug Scene," *Journal of the American Medical Association, 213: 422-425, (No. 3), July 20, 1970.*

Three physicians of the Department of Psychiatry and the Student Health Center of Stanford University report that the use of psychedelic drugs produces distortions that are experienced as strange but tolerable, even pleasant and exhilarating experiences in the majority of individuals.

In some persons a state of anxiety ranging from mild apprehension to panic occurs. The threatening situation is known as a "bad trip." It arises out of an extremely complex drug scene involving multiple drugs, unknown compounds, adulteration, contamination and deadly potentials of psychedelic agents. An ever-increasing list of new drugs leads to drug fads as the popularity of one drug gives way to that of another.

Protection of the individual from dangerous behavior (to himself or others) should be of fundamental concern in treating the bad trip, according to the three physicians. Evaluation of the patient in a quiet place is desirable. He should not be left alone.

The physician should try to find out which drug has been taken, how much was used and the approximate time it was taken. The experience of others who took the same drug should be explored in order to judge whether the reaction is due to the susceptibility of one person only. Previous efforts at treatment should be determined, especially in regard to any medication that might have been given. The fear of legal consequences often makes it difficult to gather needed information. For this reason it must be emphasized that all information will be kept confidential. Identification of any drugs should be verified by physical evidence of the drug if possible.

Observations are helpful in determining the cause of the bad trip. Hallucinogens such as LSD and mescaline generally produce dilated pupils and hyperactive reflexes. Amphetamines are apt to cause increased motor activity, excessive sweating, and a rapid pulse rate. The opiates (morphine, heroin) cause a contraction of the pupils. Marijuana causes a redness of the conjunctiva (internal portion of the eyelid and associated attachment to the eyeball), but no dilation of the pupils. Thus, the "red eye" may be a result of the smoking of marijuana.

A wide variation of mental states may be found in the person undergoing a bad trip. The range may be from mild apprehension to severe panic. With high dosage of drugs, the victim may exhibit toxic brain signs with disorientation and clouded consciousness. Illusions and hallucinations are usually present and can be highly terrifying. The victim may feel he is going to lose control and never come back. An important indicator of how severe the reaction is comes from the degree to which a person can recognize that his reaction is drug-induced and that the effects will pass. Such a person generally makes a successful recovery at the end of the experience. The absence of such an observation and understanding may indicate a severe disruption or psychosis.

Establishment of verbal contact with the patient is important. It is a fundamental rule in the management of "bad trips," and should be maintained with a minimum use of tranquilizers. If contact with reality is maintained through reassurance and repeated expression of what is real, these communications alone may be adequate treatment. In defining reality it must be explained over and over that the distortions and frightening feelings are due to the drug. Patients should be encouraged to describe their feelings and can often begin to control them rather than being overwhelmed by them. Simple repetitive statements of a concrete nature are helpful, such as: "This is a book. Feel the book." It is often helpful to a panicked bad tripper to tell him his name and that he is in a hospital, over and over.

Recovery is often of an in-and-out nature. This fact should be explained to the victim. The verbal "talkdown" with continuing reassurance and defining of reality is usually effective when given over an adequate amount of time. A physician may not have that much time. Medication may be used for a more rapid disappearance or control of symptoms. The drug most often used is chlorpromazine, the dosage of which is, of course, under control of the doctor. The value of phenothiazines may be due to their sedative effects; the three physicians of this report have found encouraging results from the use of sedating drugs.

Prolonged use of speed often results in severe depression with increased risk of suicide when the person is "brought down." A depressed patient may need hospitalization after a bad trip, but most persons can be put under the watch of a responsible person for 24 hours after they return home.

effects of drugs in the body*

Conney, A. H. "Drug Metabolism and Therapeutics," *New England Journal of Medicine,* 280: 635-660, (No. 12), March 20, 1969.

A scientist of the Wellcome Research Laboratories in Tuckahoe, New York reports that studies of the past 10 years have given dramatic evidence that *the duration and intensity of action of many drugs depend on the action of enzymes located in the liver.*

The newborn infant is more sensitive than the adult to many drugs. For this reason physicians use great care in giving drugs to infants or to an expectant mother. Barbiturates, narcotics, and other drugs cross through the placenta and may cause a deficiency of oxygen in the unborn child or may cause his death. An explanation for the sensitivity of infants to drugs lies in the fact that *newborn animals do not yet have certain enzyme systems* for the metabolism (production of chemical changes) of many drugs. The development of these enzyme systems with increasing age is accompanied by an ability to handle many drugs.

It is difficult to predict how a particular person may react to a drug. Individual differences in rates of metabolism of drugs can vary tremendously. For example, the biologic half-life of one anticoagulant drug may vary 10-fold. One patient receiving this drug maintained a

*Oliver E. Byrd, *Medical Readings on Drug Abuse,* 1970, Addison-Wesley, Reading, Mass.

high blood level for seven days; another patient had none of the drug in his blood after three days. With one antidepressant drug, the blood level in one patient was 36 times as great as that of another patient who had been given the same amount at the same time.

When two or more drugs are taken simultaneously the ability of one drug to stimulate or inhibit the action of another drug may become important. For example, it was found in animal experiments with a particular barbital drug that animals receiving another certain drug would sleep five times longer than when they received the barbital alone. It has now been documented that one drug can inhibit the metabolism of another drug in humans.

When a drug is used over a long period of time, the metabolism of other drugs may be stimulated (or depressed), and even its own metabolism may be enhanced. The stimulating effects of some drugs on their own metabolism is probably the explanation for the tolerance that occurs when a drug is given over a long time.

It is clear that many drugs affect the enzyme systems of the liver and that changes in normal metabolism of many substances occur. It is essential that the nature and importance of the multiple reactions that occur be better understood. Some persons metabolize a drug so rapidly that effective blood and tissue levels are not achieved, whereas other persons metabolize the same drug so slowly that toxic effects occur. The measurement of blood levels of any drug used by the physician is an important research necessity. There is no longer any doubt that liver enzymes are exceedingly important in respect to the effects of drugs.

multiple effects of drugs*

Bressler, R. "Combined Drug Therapy," American Journal of the Medical Sciences, 255: 89-93 (No. 2), February 1968.

The Professor of Medicine and Pharmacology at Duke University points out that *the last 20 years in medicine have seen the simultaneous use of many drugs* in the treatment of patients.

*Oliver E. Byrd, *Medical Readings on Drug Abuse,* 1970, Addison-Wesley, Reading, Mass.

Since the values or hazards of any new drug are determined through tests in which one drug alone is used, *it is unrealistic to assume that a drug will produce the same effect when used with another drug as when it is used alone.* On the contrary, one drug may markedly influence the action of another.

There are many possible actions of drugs. One of the actions is to increase *the production of enzymes* (compounds that can act on other substances) that can change the drugs to which the body is exposed. The increase of liver enzymes that can reduce the action of drugs has been observed to occur when man is exposed to a variety of drugs, pesticides, food additives and hydrocarbons in the environment that are capable of producing cancer. When a drug is broken down into some subsequent part it may be advantageous to the body where the product is less toxic than the original drug. In this case, the increase in the production of liver enzymes may lessen the effect of the drug. On the other hand, the products of drug breakdown or metabolism may equal or even exceed the toxicity of the parent drug.

Drug interactions are not limited in man to a stimulatory effect on drug metabolism or breakdown. Certain drugs can inhibit the metabolism of other drugs. Some drugs can intensify the actions of other drugs. Some drugs may stimulate or inhibit the production of enzymes, may have an effect on the absorption of other drugs, or may influence the binding of drugs to certain body tissues, or may inhibit or increase the excretion of a drug. *Many complicated effects of drugs can occur* and the complexity of possible reactions is greatly increased when more than one drug is taken simultaneously, as is often the case.

For example, Dicumerol is a drug used as an anti-coagulant for the prevention of strokes from the formation of blood clots in certain patients. When phenobarbital is used simultaneously it significantly increases the dosage of Dicumerol if protection against clotting is to be maintained. Phenobarbital and tranquilizers are often used in patients with diseases that require control of the blood clotting mechanisms, because of the associated anxiety that may be found. The combined use of drugs may result in cerebral hemorrhage and death.

Modern medicine has a vast array of drugs that can save human life, but a new *awareness is needed for their precise and proper use* in combination as well as when they are used alone.

near-fatal reaction to heroin*

Werner, Arnold. "Near-Fatal Hyperacute Reaction to Intravenously Administered Heroin," *Journal of the American Medical Association,* 207: 2277-2278, (No. 12), March 24, 1969.

A physician of the Department of Psychiatry of the Temple University School of Medicine in Philadelphia observes that *deaths from opium, heroin, and morphine (the opium alkaloids) are almost always due to the stopping of respiration.* The brain apparently becomes less sensitive to the amount of carbon dioxide in the blood and the brain centers that regulate the breathing rhythm seem likewise affected. However, in many sudden deaths of narcotic addicts the explanation has remained a mystery.

Some deaths from the injection of narcotics occur so rapidly that the needle is still in the vein when the body is found. The rapidity of such a fatal reaction does not suggest an overdosage of the drug, nor does the type of reaction of the victim lead to the same conclusion.

In this report, Dr. Werner recites the case of a man in his twenties who stopped in a service station to give himself a shot of heroin in the men's room. Dr. Werner describes the events that led to his saving of the narcotic addict as follows:

"It was a clear spring day . . . I was in my car waiting for a traffic light to change when I noticed an automobile coming out of a service station heading toward me . . . I realized the driver was slumped over the steering wheel . . . the runaway car . . . struck the side of my vehicle. I ran to the other car which was occupied by three men in addition to the driver . . . a policeman appeared and called an ambulance. The other men fled . . . on examination . . . there were no respirations, pulse could not be palpated, and heart sounds could not be heard with a stethoscope. There was no odor of alcohol. Immediate mouth-to-mouth resuscitation was begun alternating with closed-chest cardiac

*Oliver E. Byrd, *Medical Readings on Drug Abuse,* 1970, Addison-Wesley, Reading, Mass.

massage. After 5 minutes cyanosis (blueness) was less severe . . . a (heart beat) was present . . . the ambulance arrived . . . oxygen was administered . . . the man was awake, sitting up, had normal vital signs, and was responding to questions . . . the service station attendant informed (that) some blood and a burned bottle cap were found in the bathroom and that he recalled seeing the patient leave . . . immediately before the accident . . . that evening . . . the patient revealed he had taken some heroin intravenously in the service station bathroom . . . he denied being a regular user . . . said he had taken the same amount before without difficulty."

Dr. Werner concludes that an acute and temporary disturbance of the brain centers that control the rhythm of respiration would account for the complications of this case. Without artificial respiration the victim would have died.

symptoms of heroin usage

Rathod, N. H., R. de Alarcon and I. G. Thomson. "Signs of Heroin Usage Detected by Drug Users and Their Parents," Lancet, 2: 1411-1414, (No. 7531), December 30, 1967.

Three physicians of the Horsham Psychiatric Service of St. Christopher's Day Hospital in Sussex, England report a study on how you can recognize that a person is taking heroin.

Twenty heroin users between the ages of 14 and 21 years were asked to respond to a list of 38 possible signs; 20 parents of neroin addicts also cooperated in the study. The list of 38 possible signs of heroin use had been previously prepared by 12 heroin addicts and their parents who spontaneously described the observations or signs by which they were able to recognize that heroin users were under the influence of the drug.

The 20 leading signs of heroin use, as agreed upon by 50 per cent or more of *both addicts and parents,* were as follows:

	Percentage of Recognition	
Sign of Heroin Use	By Addict	By Parent
1. Wants to be left alone, may get very irritable	100	85
2. Looks dreamy and detached, seems far away	100	85
3. Does not want a proper meal	100	80
4. Blood spots clothes (pajama tops and shirts)	100	50
5. Slow and slurred speech	97	70
6. Cannot concentrate	93	75
7. Perspires	93	75
8. Rubbing of eyes, chin, and nasal areas	93	75
9. Fidgety with hands and paces up and down	93	70
10. Scratches arms and legs and areas where clothes rub	93	65
11. Unexpected absences from home (to obtain supply of heroin)	93	65
12. Sleeps out, loses motivation	93	65
13. Resents being disturbed or spoken to; avoids noise	93	65
14. Wakefulness interrupted by absences or drowsiness	93	65
15. Receives and makes frequent telephone calls (to check on supplies)	93	55
16. Posture very relaxed: lies down	87	80
17. Does not want to eat	87	70
18. Gives up organized activities	87	60

Sign of Heroin Use	Percentage of Recognition	
	By Addict	By Parent
19. Wide open and glazed eyes	80	80
20. May go to toilet to vomit	73	70

heroin overdosage and the lungs

Karliner, Joel S., Alfred D. Steinberg and M. Henry Williams, Jr. "Lung Function after Pulmonary Edema Associated with Heroin Overdosage," Archives of Internal Medicine, 124: 350-353, (No. 3), September 1969.

Three physicians of the Albert Einstein College of Medicine and the Bronx Municipal Hospital Center of New York City report *a study of the effects of heroin overdosage on the functioning of the lungs.*

It is well known to physicians that *swelling and congestion of the lung tissues may occur rapidly and may contribute to the death of a drug user who has taken an overdose of heroin.* Congestion and swelling of lung tissues may occur as late as 24 hours after the use of the drug. However, no previous studies have been reported on longer effects on lung tissues.

The three physicians studied 14 male heroin addicts who were 17 to 34 years of age.

Lung volume, vital capacity and other measures of lung functioning were performed on the subjects, all of whom showed excellent cooperation with the physicians. *Vital capacity and total lung capacity were reduced by approximately one-half in the patients who had suffered from lung swelling and congestion* because of an overdosage of heroin, as compared to normal expectancy. Ten to 12 weeks later two of the drug users had recovered to a level of only two-thirds of the predicted capacity. One patient, who suffered from an overdose of heroin but did not have swelling of lung tissue, was measured at 71 per cent of normal vital capacity and 65 per cent of expected total lung capacity.

Other laboratory tests of lung functioning confirmed the fact that significant abnormalities occur after the patient's recovery from heroin overdosage. Although slow improvement takes place the abnormalities may persist for months or longer.

The reason why lung tissue swells from heroin overdosage is not understood, but it is suspected that low oxygen content of the blood and partial failure of the left side of the heart are at fault. Lung congestion from heroin overdosage responds readily to treatment with oxygen, and it is known that the heart suffers from oxygen deficiency.

Whether or not permanent, chronic lung disease develops in heroin addicts remains an unanswered question, but *this study suggests that the repeated use of heroin may produce important obstructive lung disability eventually.*

x-ray evidence of heroin intoxication*

Stern, Wilhelm Z., Paul W. Spear and Harold G. Jacobson. "The Roentgen Findings in Acute Heroin Intoxication," American Journal of Roentgenology, Radium Therapy and Nuclear Medicine, 103: 522-532, (No. 3), July 1968.

Three physicians from the Department of Radiology and Medicine of Montefiore Hospital and Medical Center and the Department of Radiology of the Albert Einstein College of Medicine in New York City report a study of 15 patients suffering from *acute heroin intoxication.*

The *medical complications* that arise from the injection of heroin into the veins *may be divided into two categories:* 1) effects due to the heroin itself, and 2) those infections and complications associated with the non-sterile techniques of injection. The second category includes abscesses at the injection site, inflammation of adjoining body cells, inflammation of blood vessels, infections of the heart, liver and

*Oliver E. Byrd, *Medical Readings on Drug Abuse*, 1970, Addison-Wesley, Reading, Mass.

other organs of the body, tetanus, and other disorders. The first category involving the direct effects of heroin itself, includes that of heroin intoxication, or overdosage. An overdose of heroin can be rapidly fatal, or, under proper treatment, recovery can occur quite promptly.

The three physicians, all specialists in use of the x-ray, conducted their study of the 15 victims of heroin *by radiological techniques.* Twelve of the patients were hospitalized because of an overdosage of heroin; the other three patients were studied because of the presence of a serious infection related to the use of heroin.

The most striking x-ray findings in heroin addicts were in the lungs. Diffuse swelling of lung tissues, pneumonia, lung abscess, partial collapse of a lung and fluid were found in and around the lung tissues. One of the victims died within several hours; another died after eight days. Six of the patients showed x-ray clearing of the lungs within 24 to 48 hours; four of the victims improved after 4 to 6 days. Two other victims needed three to six weeks before there was x-ray evidence of control of disease.

The symptoms of heroin overdosage consist of a comatose or stuporous condition, depressed respiration, and constricted pupils. The sound of fluid in the lungs, bloody sputum, and other symptoms may be present also.

Emergency treatment consists of the intravenous injection of 5 mg. of nalorphine hydrochloride (nalline) which generally controls the respiratory depression and brings significant recovery within 24 to 48 hours. It is the respiratory depression and diminished ventilation that leads to a deficiency of oxygen, which in turn is related to an increased permeability of the blood vessels in the lungs and swelling of the lung tissues.

Abscesses in various parts of the body due to needle infections may be revealed by x-ray also. Broken needle fragments are sometimes found. Other complications of heroin usage may be detected at times.

symptoms of narcotic addiction in the newborn

Mims, LeRoy C. and Harris D. Riley, Jr. "The Narcotic Withdrawal Syndrome in the Newborn Infant," *Journal of the Oklahoma State Medical Association, 62: 411-412, (No. 9), September 1969.*

Two physicians express their concern for *the newborn narcotic addict* in an editorial published in a state medical journal. The two doctors observe that in recent years there has been a remarkable increase on a national scale in the use of narcotics and the development of addiction in females of childbearing age.

During pregnancy the unborn child becomes a drug addict if the mother-to-be continues her narcotic addiction. At birth the newborn infant is suddenly shut off from his supply of narcotics which he has been receiving from the mother's bloodstream. *Within hours the infant will be suffering withdrawal symptoms* that may threaten his life.

At the University of Oklahoma Medical Center a newly-born infant began to develop narcotic withdrawal symptoms within 24 hours. Physicians were able to document the fact that the mother of the infant was addicted to morphine and were alert to the possibility that the baby might need treatment for withdrawal symptoms.

The baby began to develop *extreme irritability,* suffered from *diarrhea, nausea and vomiting.* The infant *cried* frequently and for prolonged periods of time in a *high-pitched, shrill tone of voice.* Other symptoms included *yawning and sneezing, tremors* (tremblings and shakings), *flushed skin, profuse sweating and fever.* Sometimes profound *shock, convulsions* and *death* may occur, although in this case the baby was treated promptly because of the anticipated reactions and recovered satisfactorily.

Failure to recognize narcotic withdrawal symptoms in the newborn baby with consequent failure to render appropriate medical treatment *means that approximately 95 per cent of the infants* addicted to drugs at birth *will die.* Thus, there is *an overwhelming risk of death* for the baby if the condition is not recognized. In one study it was found that of 37 addicted babies who were not treated, 33 died.

A treatment program for the addicted baby should be available and put into operation as soon as symptoms of withdrawal begin to occur. A preventive program for the baby during pregnancy is usually not possible since it is generally advised that no withdrawal of the pregnant mother should be attempted after the seventh month of pregnancy.

Paregoric and chlorpromazine are reported by the physicians as being the most effective drugs for treatment of the addicted infant. Precise dosages and time intervals are given in the orginal article cited above, but *it may take three to seven weeks before all drugs can be discontinued.* The physicians observe that *long-range planning may mean the baby should be taken from his mother* by adoption or he is apt to grow up in a world of addicts with every likelihood of becoming permanently addicted in adult life.

10
poisonings

Children are the principal victims of poisonings, but the non-lethal effects often go unrecognized. Different poisons call for different first aid measures and different medical treatments, but there are certain general principles of removal, absorption and dilution that have been proven by time and experience to have value if applied swiftly before spread of the poison throughout the body.

Insecticides and other chemicals in the environment have increased the likelihood of accidental poisonings among agricultural workers, children, and even the general public. It is likely that the hazard of poisonings will never be completely controlled in our society.

health effects of insecticides

Ecobichon, D. J. "Chlorinated hydrocarbon insecticides: Recent animal data of potential significance for man," Journal of the Canadian Medical Association, 103: 711-716, (No. 7), October 10, 1970.

A member of the Faculty of Medicine, Dalhousie University, in Halifax, Nova Scotia reports that of all the insecticides contributing to the pollution problem, *the chlorinated hydrocarbons are* by far the worst offenders. Originally they were thought to be the ideal insecticide because they were highly toxic to insects and had little risk for humans. Over one billion pounds of DDT alone are available at present to the atmosphere.

However, because *the chemicals are so stable, they accumulate in the fat of animals and man until they may reach concentrations of 80,000 to ten million times.* Herein lies the hazard to mankind.

Acute poisoning in humans is rare and usually involves young children who have accidentally swallowed DDT or one of its derivatives.

The symptoms of acute poisoning include vomiting, diarrhea, dizziness, rapid heart rate, shallow, rapid breathing, difficult breathing, abdominal swelling, unconsciousness and convulsions.

Chronic poisoning with large amounts of insecticide causes death of liver cells, degeneration of the kidney, blood disorders, small hemorrhages in the lungs and heart muscle and swelling of the brain and spinal cord with nervous impairment.

Long time exposure to small or moderate amounts of chlorinated hydrocarbons results in little evidence of illness. The explanation seems to lie in the fact that the insecticide is rapidly stored in fat and is thus removed from the remainder of body tissues. The potential danger arises when for one reason or another the fat is used for energy and the insecticide is released again. Signs of poisoning may be observed if the amounts released are large enough.

The newly-born are highly sensitive to insecticide poisoning at levels far below those that would be needed to injure adults. The reasons are thought to be that the newly born have little fat in which to store the chemical, there are few liver enzymes available to destroy it, the kidneys are still immature and not fully developed and natural barriers in the body to spreading of the chemical are not well developed.

Various endocrine changes are related to the action of the chlorinated hydrocarbons. DDT is similar in structural configuration to the synthetic estrogen diethylstilbestrol. The estrogenic activity of this compound has been investigated and is thought to be involved in the decreased thickness of eggshells in birds because of interference with the use of calcium.

Liver enzymes are increased and various structural changes of the liver are induced by the insecticides being discussed.

It is not yet known if DDT and its compounds can cause cancer. Mice given DDT did not develop cancer, but in each successive generation thereafter for five generations there was an increase in the amount of leukemia and malignant tumors. The insecticides aldrin and heptachlor, however, have been shown to cause a four-fold increase in liver cancers.

In humans the *amount of insecticides found in fatty tissues is rising* and the average yearly intake of DDT and its derivatives is reported to be about 50 mg. 90 per cent comes from food. To date, however, according to Dr. Ecobichon, there appears to be little risk of poisoning of the average populations. Possibly *the greatest danger is in those groups involved in spraying of orchards and crops or handling the sprayed materials.* These people do harbor high fat levels of insecticide. No adverse effects are observed unless illness, surgery, stress, or dieting uses up the body fat and releases the chemical. *Female agricultural workers and the wives of farmers during pregnancy* would be in most hazard in the agricultural groups because the insecticide might be liberated from fat, and transferred to the unborn baby as well as appearing in the mothers' milk to the ultimate handicap of the child.

pesticide poisoning in children

DePalma, Arthur E., Donald S. Kwalick and Nathan Zukerberg. "Pesticide Poisoning in Children," Journal of the American Medical Association, 211: 1979-1981, (No. 12), March 23, 1970.

Three physicians of the Department of Pediatrics of St. James Hospital in Newark, New Jersey report the cases of an 8-year old sister and a 5-year old brother who were treated in the emergency room because their mother had given a dark liquid from a jar in the refrigerator, which she thought to be coffee, to her daughter and son. The daughter drank the liquid and the son spit it out. The sister died and the brother lived. The substance they drank was a pesticide containing parathion, chlordane, and dimpylate. The highest blood and tissue levels of these pesticides that have ever been reported were found in the children.

The sister died, despite the most intensive and adequate medical care that could be provided. The young brother, despite the onset of convulsions and coma, as well as respiratory failure, did live, after the most intensive medical treatment.

The death of liver cells in the case of the sister was judged to be due to parathion, rather than the two other substances that were in the liquid consumed. Although it is unlikely that the boy will suffer chronic liver damage, he will be observed medically for many years.

The emergency treatment of these two children poisoned with pesticide consisted of two important measures: 1) *artificial respiration and 2) emptying the stomach of its contents.*

After that, medical treatment was provided to stop the convulsions and to counteract the other effects of the pesticide contents with atropine sulfate every five minutes. Still other measures were used which were successful in the case of the boy, but unsuccessful in the case of the girl because of the massive dose of the pesticide in the latter.

The onset of symptoms of abdominal pain, heart stoppage, respiratory failure and loss of consciousness, as well as convulsions, was rapid. Symptoms progressed to severe conditions at a rapid rate also.

The material the children had consumed had been used to exterminate cockroaches three days earlier. The left-over materials had been carelessly saved by the parents.

immediate treatment of poisoning

Phansalkar, S. V. and L. Emmett Holt, Jr. "Observations on the immediate treatment of treatment of poisoning," Journal of Pediatrics, 72: 683-685 (No. 5), May 1968.

Two members of the Department of Pediatrics of the New York University School of Medicine observe that the urgent and immediate treatment of poisoning should be directed toward *reducing the amount of poison that is absorbed* in the stomach and intestines.

It is ideal emergency treatment if the poison can be removed by lavage (washing out the stomach) or by vomiting. The next best procedure is to give some substance to the victim that can be swallowed and which will absorb the poison and thus prevent its passage from the stomach into the intestines or into the circulatory system.

Aspirin is the most common cause of poisoning in young children.

Activated charcoal has been recommended by physicians as one of the most absorbent substances which is effective against a wide variety of poisons. Charcoal is effective as soon as it is swallowed and can be safely used as a home remedy.

In this study, animals that had received no charcoal were given 100 grains of aspirin. It was found that their blood levels of this substance rose rapidly within 30 minutes and continued to rise for several hours. When charcoal was given there was a sharp reduction of absorption of the aspirin. When as much as 90 grams of charcoal were given there was no blood evidence of the absorption of aspirin at all. When the charcoal was given even as late as one-half hour after the swallowing of aspirin, the rise in blood level of the substance was halted immediately. It appears that *charcoal is helpful even if given some time after the aspirin poisoning.*

In a 70-pound child who received 35 grains of aspirin, it was found that *small doses of charcoal were not sufficient to stop absorption, but when the dosage of charcoal was increased it was adequate to prevent absorption of the drug. The amount of charcoal can be increased safely and it is effective for aspirin poisoning immediately after it is swallowed.*

The use of ipecac to induce vomiting was found to be ineffective in dogs when given by mouth, and it cannot be depended upon in children, for *as many as 12 per cent of children will not vomit within 30 minutes after the drug.* Charcoal, in contrast, is effective at once.

Four available preparations of activated charcoal are known as Darco G 60, Nuchar CN, Norit A, and Norit U.S.P. XVII. Directions for use of the substances should be followed.

In conclusion, *activated charcoal appears to be one of the best substances for immediate use in aspirin poisoning.*

poison accidents in childhood

Verhulst, Henry L. and John J. Crotty. "Childhood Poisoning Accidents," Journal of the American Medical Association, 203: 1049-1050, (No. 12) March 18, 1968.

Information from the Poison Control Branch of the Public Health Service, as reported by a physician and his associate, indicate that between one-half million to two million American children accidentally swallow some poisonous substance every year. As a result approximately 500 children under the age of five die from accidental poisoning.

Ninety per cent of the medical reports to the National Clearinghouse involve children under the age of five who have swallowed poisonous materials found in or around the house. In about one-half the cases, the substances swallowed are medicines, and in the other half of the cases other household products are swallowed.

One-fourth of the total poisonings are caused by swallowing aspirin. Cleaning and polishing agents (15%), pesticides (6%), turpentine paints (5%), petroleum products (5%) and cosmetics (6%) are the household products in addition to aspirin that are most commonly swallowed by children.

Most poisoning accidents occur to children between the ages of 18 and 24 months. The younger children tend to swallow household products, and the older children tend to swallow medicines. Accidents happen most frequently in the kitchen, bedroom and bathroom.

Two-thirds of the substances swallowed were not in their customary place of storage. When products are shifted to soft-drink bottles, cups, and glasses, the chances of accidental swallowing by children are greatly increased.

In the United States there are now *approximately 550 poison control centers* that *can give information to physicians on poisons* and their treatment on an emergency basis. The first such poison control center was established in Chicago in 1953. The physician cannot know the toxic ingredients of every substance, but these poison control centers have this information, along with the recommended medical treatment.

The National Clearinghouse for the Poison Control Centers now tabulates information on about 85,000 cases of poisonings each year.

A *Guide for Teaching Poison Prevention in Kindergarten* has been prepared to instruct the preschooler on poison prevention. The purpose is to teach responsibility of the kindergarten child for younger brothers and sisters and to educate parents to the nature of the problem.

Primary treatment involves the induction of vomiting. The use of syrup of Ipecac for this purpose has become increasingly popular. It can be kept in the homes for this emergency. [Note comment on this subject in preceding article, however.— Ed.]

household poisonings

Conference on Therapy. "Household Poisonings," The American Journal of Medicine, 6: 237-46, (No. 2), February 1949.

A conference on household poisonings by members of the Departments of Pharmacology and of Medicine of Cornell University and the New York Hospital brought to light certain facts about this problem.

The major proportion of household poisonings occur in children. The drugs and chemicals involved in these poisonings cover a very wide field. In one report listing 158 cases of fatal poisonings in a five-year period in children under five years of age in New York State there were forty-five different substances listed.

About half of all the cases of fatal poisonings in this group, namely, 75 of the 158, were due to strychnine. There was no close second in the entire list. The remaining 83 cases were caused by forty-four different substances.

A telephone call was received from a pediatrician regarding the possibility of poisoning from matches. The child was playing with a box of safety matches and chewed off the tips. The problem related to the possibility of phosophorus poisoning. To get into difficulties from that adventure the child would have had to consume the box rather than the matches.

The friction match which can be struck anywhere was originally tipped with yellow phosphorus. Fifteen or 20 tips might provide a fatal dose of phosphorus. But in the safety match the phosphorus is on the striking surface of the box and even this in present-day matches no longer contains the highly toxic yellow phosphorus but the unabsorbable red phosphorus. The latter is relatively nontoxic, although some contamination with yellow phosphorus is a source of danger. *Even the ordinary match, which may be struck anywhere, is now relatively innocuous because the nontoxic red phosphorus has replaced the yellow phosphorus.*

Camphorated oil is sometimes mistaken for castor oil; it might be well, therefore, to know something about the toxicity of camphorated oil. *Camphor is a convulsant but it is very rapidly eliminated, so that even after a fairly violent convulsion the individual is likely to recover.*

Infants and children seem to have little trouble in getting hold of a bottle or can of kerosene or gasoline. Also, they do not seem to have any particular aversion to drinking it. A considerable number of cases of poisoning are encountered. There are recoveries from as much as 125 cc. of kerosene and deaths from as little as 30 cc. *The course of kerosene poisoning is very rapid.* Effects appear within a few minutes with gastrointestinal symptoms (vomiting, diarrhea, abdominal cramps) and central nervous system symptoms (coma, convulsions). About 5 to 10 percent of the patients die; this takes place in less than 24 hours. The remainder seem to recover completely and fairly promptly. It is fairly safe to assume that the patient who is still alive on the day after a dose of kerosene is likely to recover. The lungs seem to be involved in a large proportion of the cases. Such a case may be mistaken for one of primary pneumonia. It is not certain how the lungs become involved, whether by excretion of the volatile agent through the lungs or by aspiration during vomiting.

The extermination of household pests provides a rich and varied source of household poisons.

Dry cleaning fluids and stain removers are very common household poisons. The more common ones represent carbon tetrachloride, or mixtures of carbon tetrachloride, solvent naphtha, turpentine, benzine, gasoline, and kerosene. Cases of poisoning result both from the inhalation of vapors as well as from ingestion. A woman who had cleaned a dress with carbon tetrachloride in the bathroom, a small space without ventilation, succumbed to the fumes of this compound.

Black shoe dye often contains nitrobenzene. It is a potent poison. As little as 1 cc. may prove fatal although 30 cc. have been survived. It is readily absorbed through the skin of an infant's foot as well as by inhalation. It causes bizarre symptoms involving the gastrointestinal tract, the central nervous system, and the viscera.

The laxative known as Ex-Lax, which contains phenolphthalein, is another source of trouble. The usual story when children are brought in is that they have consumed from twelve to twenty-four of these chocolates.

Many of the preparations containing poisons to which children are exposed in the home fail to provide the physician with a clue to the essential chemical.

leading poisonings in children

Chun, L. T. "Accidental Poisoning in Children," Hawaii Medical Journal, 11: 83-87, (No. 2), November-December 1951.

L. T. Chun, M.D., of Honolulu, reports on a study of accidental poisoning in 221 cases among children admitted for hospital treatment over a five-year period. Fifty-nine different poisons were encountered in this series of cases. Twice as many boys were poisoned as girls. The age of greatest frequency was two years, with almost all of the cases occurring between one and three years. Approximately one percent of the children died from the poisoning.

The time between poisoning and medical aid ranged from about one-half hour to one hour. In most cases the exact amount of poison consumed was unknown.

The numbers of children poisoned by the ten leading types of poison involved are given in the following table:

Rank	Poison	Number
1	Kerosene	69
2	Arsenic	17
3	Oil of eucalyptus	13
4	Phenolphthalein	7
5	Pine oil	7
6	Barbiturates	7
7	Butter fish (spoiled)	7
8	Salicylates	6
9	Camphorated oil	5
10	Rubbing alcohol	4
11	Turpentine	4

aspirin poisoning

Gardner, Emily. *"Aspirin Poisoning," Virginia Medical Monthly, 80: 147-51, (No. 3), March 1953.*

Emily Gardner, M.D., of Richmond, Virginia, states that aspirin poisoning in children *may be very serious.* Dr. Gardner states that infants and children seem peculiarly susceptible to relatively small amounts of aspirin. She reviews 77 cases of poisoning from this drug which have been reported in the medical literature within recent years. In this group there were eleven deaths.

Symptoms of aspirin poisoning may not appear for twelve to twenty-four hours after toxic amounts of the drug have been swallowed. When given in divided doses there is often an accumulative effect, as symptoms may not appear for one to four days.

Difficult breathing, caused by an acidosis, is a constant symptom. This abnormal respiration continues until the acidosis has been corrected or the patient dies of respiratory failure. Other symptoms frequently found are vomiting, an acetone odor to the breath, irritability, restlessness, cyanosis or pallor, semiconsciousness or stupor, profuse sweating, dehydration, often fever of a high degree, and sometimes convulsions and abdominal pain. Other symptoms may also be present.

Treatment depends upon the time when the patient reaches the physician. *The stomach should be emptied and large quantities of fluid given the patient.* The patient first undergoes an alkalosis but later progresses to a second stage of compensated acidosis. These conditions must be counterbalanced by medical treatment, and vitamin K and vitamin C are advised to help control bleeding.

The lethal dose of aspirin for human beings is not exactly known. Sick children who are taking little food or fluids appear to be especially susceptible to aspirin poisoning. *Parents should be especially warned against the dangers of overdosage with aspirin that has been sweetened or otherwise made attractive to children.* Generally a safe dose of aspirin for children is one grain of the drug, per year of age, every four hours.

lead poisoning in children

Ellington, Preston D. "Lead Poisoning in Children," Journal of the Medical Association of Georgia, 43: 33-35, (No. 1), January 1954.

Preston D. Ellington, M.D., of Augusta, Georgia, says that epidemics and sporadic cases of lead poisoning have been reported for a number of years and that the sources of the lead involved in such poisonings are numerous.

Water supplies conducted through lead pipes have been an important source of community poisonings. The use of lead-containing bath powders have caused lead poisoning in many infants and mothers. The perverted appetite of the child has accounted for the eating of lead from the siderails of newly painted cribs and painted toys. Other sources of lead compounds include painted plaster and paint flakes from toys, furniture, and windowsills. Lead poisoning is often caused by the use of discarded battery storage cases. The battery cases are impregnated with particles of lead sulphide which are vaporized when the casings are burned. These discarded cases serve as a source of fuel and heat during times of family economic distress but may lead to lead poisoning.

The symptoms of lead poisoning in children vary with the duration and intensity of the exposure and with the susceptibility of the child. *One of the earliest symptoms to be noted is a change in the disposition. The child may become restless at night, be irritable and peevish during the waking hours, and complain of pain in the upper center of the abdomen, with indefinite pains in the joints and muscles, especially in the legs.* The appetite usually becomes poor. As the disease progresses, the abdominal pains are more severe and the child may become constipated.

Perhaps the most dramatic manifestation of lead poisoning and, at the same time, one which is of the most serious significance, is the development of acute mental change. Convulsions from inflammation of the brain due to lead poisoning may be very persistent, with a tendency to recur and with a high mortality rate.

Dr. Ellington reports the case of a fourteen-month-old child who developed acute lead poisoning from the inhalation of fumes generated by the burning of battery casings in an open hearth for about three months preceding the illness of the child.

throat damage from corrosives

Brigham, Dwight, and Herman M. Jahr. "Stenosis of the Esophagus Due to Ingestion of Corrosives," Nebraska State Medical Journal, 38: 14-17, (No. 1), January 1953.

Drs. Dwight Brigham and Herman M. Jahr, of Omaha, Nebraska, report that although deaths from the drinking of corrosives such as Drano, drain-pipe cleaners, ammonia, lye, and Sani-Flush are not frequent, the illness resulting from a consumption of such products is substantial.

Corrosive esophagitis, as this condition is called, occurs primarily in small children from the age of one to three years. The condition is sometimes seen in adults who have tried to commit suicide.

The corrosive agents most frequently encountered are those alkaline substances that can be readily obtained from the local grocer and are found in most homes.

Three distinct symptom periods can be observed in this type of injury. The immediate symptom is pain. A few hours later, obstruction of the throat occurs because of swelling and inflammation. The patient is usually not even able to swallow his own saliva. These early symptoms disappear over a period of the first week, usually within the first two or three days.

A second period then occurs in which the symptoms are either very mild or nonexistent. This is a period of healing of the ulcerated areas. It begins within the first week after the caustic substance has been swallowed and lasts for approximately two to four weeks.

The third period is one of fibrous tissue replacement which, over a period of a few days or weeks, produces progressive pain on swallowing. If the condition is not treated at this time it ultimately results in complete obstruction of the esophagus due to the formation of fibrous scar tissue.

Special diagnostic procedures include the x-ray examination and the use of the esophagoscope for examination of the damaged tissues. However, this latter procedure is apt to be hazardous, especially during the first month after a burn. Usually diagnosis can be made without the use of these special procedures.

After the original swelling of the mouth and throat has subsided, which is usually by the fourth or fifth day, dilation of the esophagus must be started and increased daily until a clear passage has been established. The instrument used to secure this dilation is known as a bougie: it should be kept in the esophagus for about thirty minutes before withdrawal on any single day. Gradually the number of dilatations will diminish but should be continued into the second year of treatment, although at this time it is possible that only three or four dilatations may be necessary. Often this procedure should be continued for the ensuing two years.

11
internal injuries

Even for the physician the recognition of internal injuries may be difficult. The multiple internal structures, tissues and organs that may be damaged in an accident are apt to give evidence of injury in indirect ways, and it cannot be expected that the first aider will be competent to judge their nature in specific terms. On the other hand, the possibility of multiple injuries and internal damage must always be considered in any accident.

To suspect a spinal injury may cause a first aider to take those protective measures against movement and transportation that can prevent further serious damage. Suspicion of internal bleeding may lead the person rendering first aid to more rapid access to medical services and hospital facilities. In any event, respect for the possibility of greater damage in an injured person can be expected to make the first aider more able in his handling of emergencies.

injuries to the spine

Ashworth, J. "Spinal Injuries and Fractures," British Medical Journal, 4: 414-15, (No. 5680), November 15, 1969.

A consultant orthopedic surgeon from the Darlington and Northallerton Hospitals in Yorkshire, England reports that *most cases of damage to the spinal cord are caused by an accident in a motor vehicle.* Such accidents are occurring with greater frequency than ever before.

Injuries to the spine may be classified as stable or unstable, and it is invariably in the unstable injuries that damage to the cord occurs. If cord damage does not occur at the time of the accident, it is still possible for damage to occur during extrication of the person from the vehicle or during transportation to the hospital, particularly if the person is unconscious.

The *diagnosis of a spinal injury* at the roadside can be a difficult problem. If the person is conscious he may *complain of pain over a segment of the spine.* Neurological damage may be indicated if he is unable to move one or more limbs or if he has *sensory disturbances in either the arms or the legs.* The presence of *an abrasion on the top of the skull* may denote injury from a vertical force, thus causing a possible *burst fracture of the spine in the neck area.*

With the exception of injuries in the neck region of the spine, any neurological damage usually occurs at the time of impact. Hence there is not much that can be done at the site of the accident that will affect the ultimate prognosis.

In the neck region, however, recurrence of a dislocation may take place during movement of the victim. Treatment at the roadside may therefore have a considerable effect on recovery from such injuries.

Many victims with neck injuries may also have severe head injuries, and may be unconscious or unable to give any clear indication of symptoms. But *if there is any suspicion of injury to the neck, the affected part should be immobilized.*

Immobilization of the neck is a relatively simple and effective procedure. The basic principle is to *prevent any bending movements* of the neck. This may be done adequately with *any form of neck collar which fits under the jaw and thus prevents it from sagging forward. A simple neck collar may be made from stiff cardboard, covered with cloth* for comfort, and fastened with a piece of gauze. The collar does not have to be pulled tight. The person can then be moved more safely.

Securing the victim onto a board of some kind also helps to immobilize injured parts, facilitates transportation, and may help problems of resuscitation or airway control to be overcome more easily.

injuries to the neck

Skultety, F. Miles. "Treatment of Cervical Spine Injuries," Nebraska State Medical Journal, 53: 3-5, (No. 1), January 1968.

A neurosurgeon of the University of Nebraska College of Medicine observes that any situation which subjects the body to violent motion, such as an automobile accident, may cause injury to the cervical (neck) spine. It is wise to consider that *any person with a head injury may possibly have a neck fracture.*

Fractures of the vertebral column of the neck can and do occur without damage to the spinal nerve cord, and *it is important to handle neck injury patients carefully* to prevent such an injury if it has not already occurred. On the Nebraska Neurosurgical Service, Dr. Skultety says *it is mandatory that x-rays of the cervical spine be obtained on all patients with head injuries.* These films are the first ones taken. If no fracture or dislocation is seen, then the patient can be safely moved about for other diagnostic procedures and treatment.

Only well-trained persons should attempt to move a person suspected of having a neck injury.

Unconscious (unresponsive) patients are usually transported in a semi-prone position, which helps keep the airway open and tends to prevent aspiration of fluid into the lungs. However, *an accident victim with a neck fracture should be transported in a supine position with sandbags, or some other kind of support on each side of the head.* Narcotics or *sedatives should never be given* to anyone with a cervical spine injury or head injury because of the resultant respiratory depression. In the ambulance a trained person should ride with the neck-fracture victim to provide respiratory assistance or suction if it is necessary. If a halter head traction apparatus is available it can be used during transportation.

In the hospital, the victim with an injury to the cervical spinal cord may have a temporary (or permanent) paralysis of all four limbs. These patients may have respiratory difficulties because the rib and abdominal muscles are not functioning properly. Breathing is almost entirely with the diaphragm. Two other dangers may arise: paralytic ileus (obstruction of the intestines due to paralysis) and gastro-intestinal hemorrhage. The bleeding is assumed to result from an ulceration that is associated with injury to the central nervous system ("Cushing's ulcer").

first aid for spinal cord injuries

Perret, George. "The Emergency Treatment of Spinal-Cord Injuries," Journal of the Iowa State Medical Society, 47: 252-56 (No. 5), May 1957.

George Perret, M.D., Associate Professor of Neurosurgery at the State University of Iowa College of Medicine, says that the outcome of spinal cord injuries may well depend upon the manner in which the patient is handled and transported at the scene of the accident.

If the patient is conscious, the diagnosis of a spinal cord injury can be made from the patient's statement that he is unable to feel or move his arms or legs. If the patient is unconscious, then he should be presumed to have suffered a spinal cord injury as well as a brain injury, and that assumption should be maintained until the diagnosis can be cleared.

If an unconscious patient moves all of his extremities spontaneously, there is little likelihood of his having received a spinal cord injury. However, if on examination he is found to be using his diaphragm but not his intercostal muscles for respiration, then one must assume that a spinal cord injury is present. The reflexes may be depressed as the result of cord injury as well as of brain injury. The patient should be kept in a flat, neutral position, preferably on his back or abdomen, if he is found in such a position. His legs should be extended, and his head and neck should be straightened in the axis of the rest of his body and, at the same time, kept in a position which does not interfere with his respiration. From his head to his pelvis, however, no part of his spine should be flexed or hyperextended. In the presence of a spinal injury, any degree of flexion or hyperextension may aggravate the wound and change reversible damage into an irreversible injury.

Clearance of the upper respiratory passages may be lifesaving since the impairment of respiration is frequently caused by an accumulation of mucus, vomitus or blood in the comatose patient.

One should never consider using a passenger car for transporting a patient suspected of having a spinal cord injury, for obviously he would need to be flexed when lifted through the door of such a vehicle. An ambulance should be called.

The ambulance stretcher should be put flat on the ground next to and parallel to the patient. A canvas stretcher should be avoided, for the patient's back would sag through it. A wide, flat board, a sheet of plywood or a door will serve admirably as a makeshift stretcher. If the patient is lying on his abdomen, he should be rolled onto the stretcher, or rolled onto his back and lifted to the stretcher. Four persons are needed for the job, and they must work in close cooperation to hold the patient straight. One person should hold the head and neck in the axis of the body; the second should hold the chest and upper extremities flat and straight; the third should hold the abdomen and pelvis; and the fourth should hold the lower extremities. All of their movements should be synchronized so that the patient will be moved in a stiff, boardlike fashion. At the same time, some traction should be exerted upon the feet and upon the head. The patient should then be brought to a hospital where adequate first aid and emergency treatment can be given.

At no time should the patient's head be lifted so that he may drink a glass of water or smoke a cigarette, for such a movement may be followed by severe spinal complications.

should pregnant women wear seat belts?

Crosby, Warren M. "Does it Make Sense for a Pregnant Woman to Wear a Seat Belt?" Emergency Medicine, 1: 22-23, (No. 4), May 1969.

A physician of the University of Oklahoma reports that he has been receiving reports from the California State Highway Patrol on all rural automobile accidents involving pregnant women. He now has complete records on 200 women. Data were secured from families, hospitals and physicians.

Of the 200 pregnant women, 178 were not using seat belts at the time of the accident. Primary reasons for not using the seat belts were forgetfulness, being uncomfortable and being fearful that the seat belt might injure the unborn baby or the mother in case of an accident.

Among the pregnant women who were not using a seat belt at the time of the accident, *eight died from their injuries and none of the babies survived* death of the mothers. In addition, *six other babies were born dead* because of separation of the placenta, maternal shock or other unknown cause. *Thus eight mothers and 14 babies died when seat belts were not used.*

Among the 22 pregnant women who were using seat belts, no deaths to the mothers occurred and only one child was born dead. Only a few of the mothers in this group *suffered any injuries.*

Dr. Crosby, in reviewing the medical literature, found reports on 89 more pregnant women who were involved in automobile accidents. Of this number 66 were not wearing seat belts and *six died, and all six of their babies died.* There were no deaths among the 23 women who were using a seat belt, although there were more deaths of the babies than in the California series.

Pregnant women seem to be more reluctant to use seat belts than most other people, and the major reason given is fear of injury to the unborn baby or to self. Dr. Crosby points out that the *greatest hazard to the unborn baby is the death of the mother,* that seat belts prevent many fatal injuries, and that *pregnant women should use seat belts* and should use them properly, across the upper thighs rather than over the pregnant uterus. The combination shoulder harness and lap belt should improve the survival chances of both the mother and the unborn child.

when the pregnant woman is hurt

Buchsbaum, Herbert J. "When a Pregnant Woman Gets Hurt," Emergency Medicine, 1: 20-23, (No. 4), May 1969.

An assistant professor of obstetrics and gynecology of the Downstate Medical Center in Brooklyn and the State University of New York observes that *pregnant women of today* participate freely in the driving of automobiles, work activities, and other endeavors until late in pregnancy, and as a consequence *are involved in many more accidents and injuries than in former years.*

When a pregnant woman is injured *there are two lives at stake* rather than one. This fact can complicate both diagnosis and treatment.

The likelihood of injury to the unborn baby increases with the age of the fetus. Early in pregnancy the fetus is protected by the bony pelvis and the buffering effect of the amniotic fluid. It can also withstand a greater degree of fall in blood pressure and insufficiency of oxygen. Near the time of childbirth the unborn baby is especially vulnerable to hemorrhage or blood loss that affects the mother. The mother's body is protected at the expense of the fetus. Because the mother's blood volume is greatly increased during pregnancy she can withstand a considerable loss of blood, but the unborn baby cannot. Thus, in hemorrhage of the mother it is important to use whole blood transfusion so that both fluid volume and red blood cells can be restored rapidly.

In *penetrating abdominal wounds,* effects on the mother are apt to be *less* than in a non-pregnant woman because as the pregnant uterus expands it displaces more vital abdominal organs into a smaller space and tends to absorb the energy of a bullet or other missile that penetrates the abdomen. Dr. Buchsbaum reports there have been no maternal deaths in pregnancy from gunshot wounds of the abdomen since 1912.

Priorities of treatment in pregnancy are the same as in other cases. Breathing must be sustained, hemorrhage must be controlled, shock must be treated. However, vasopressors (substances that constrict blood vessels and thereby raise the blood pressure) should not be used to treat shock during pregnancy. This is because such drugs shut down the blood supply to the unborn baby.

According to Dr. Buchsbaum *the motility of the digestive tract is reduced in pregnancy and injury reduces it further.* As a consequence a tube should be used to empty the stomach in all serious or abdominal injuries during pregnancy. If blood is found in the material removed from the stomach it may be an important clue to internal bleeding.

Any contaminated wound during pregnancy should be treated with tetanus immunization if there is doubt about the victim's immunity. Tetanus antitoxin may be advisable also. Neither of these substances has any harmful effects on the unborn baby.

X-rays are important in the diagnosis of injuries, *but in pregnancy they must be used with caution.* It has not been clearly established how much radiation will damage an unborn baby. Even low doses may be hazardous. However, x-ray examination of the arms, legs, and chest of the mother may be done without hazard, if the abdomen or fetus is properly shielded from radiation. The real *danger lies in x-raying the abdomen.*

Some physicians have inserted needles into the abdomen to see if there is internal bleeding, but Dr. Buchsbaum recommends against this procedure because the needle may not even reach the area where blood is apt to collect and intestinal loops of the bowel may be penetrated by the needle. He therefore feels that this diagnostic technique should not be used on pregnant women.

The white-blood-cell count in pregnancy may be very confusing to a physician. Counts of 20,000 to 30,000 are ordinarily considered as a sure sign of rupture of the spleen or liver in any injury, but in late pregnancy the count may go as high as 25,000 without any injury. Thus, in a pregnant woman studies of the white blood cells may be confusing.

If surgery on the mother is necessary it should be known that fairly extensive operations can be performed without disturbing the pregnancy. Even in the period after operation a baby may be delivered normally without ill effect on the mother. About the only time a Cesarian operation should be done on the injured mother occurs when there are pelvic fractures and fractures of a vertebra and the patient seems about to deliver her baby.

If an injured pregnant woman is placed on her back, especially if she is unconscious or in shock, the pregnant uterus may press the blood vessels against the spinal cord and shut off or cut down on the venous return of blood to the heart. The result is a sudden, drastic fall in blood pressure, which disappears as soon as the patient is turned on her side rather than her back. A possible serious effect of compression of the inferior vena cava (the main vein returning blood to the heart from the lower part of the body) is the increase in pressure in the veins below the point of compression. This increased pressure in the veins may cause more bleeding from any injuries to the leg or pelvic areas.

The pregnant woman should be alerted to the use of more care in everything she does. Obviously, the driver of an automobile, with a steering wheel in her lap, is in greater danger of an abdominal injury in case of accident, than a passenger. The pregnant woman should limit her driving as much as possible. She should also be encouraged to use a seat belt.

seat belt injuries

Porter, Samuel D. and Edward W. Green. "Seat Belt Injuries," Archives of Surgery, 96: 242-246 (No. 2), February 1968.

Two surgeons of the University Hospital at Iowa City report that *occasionally an injury due to the wearing of a seat belt is seen.*

Various types of abdominal injuries have been reported, including rupture of the spleen or liver, lacerations or tears of the pancreas, small intestine and large bowel or rupture of the abdominal aorta (large artery descending to the lower part of the body) as well as fractures of the lumbar spine (involving the lower back).

case histories

1 *A 21-year-old man who experienced a head-on collision* was wearing a lap-type seat belt. Thirty minutes later he was in the emergency room with a chief complaint of abdominal pain. He had an obvious fracture of the right upper arm and contusions over the lower abdomen. He went into profound shock. At surgery it was found that he had ruptured his intestine and colon, although it had been suspected before surgery that he had ruptured his spleen. After surgical repair and six weeks in the hospital he recovered.

2 *A 16-year-old boy was riding as a passenger* in the front seat when the driver side-swiped another car. The boy was wearing a seat belt. In the hospital 45 minutes later he was found to have a fractured spinal vertebra. Later he developed abdominal pain. At surgery an abdominal muscle was found to be cut apart and there was an associated rupture of the intestine. His recovery followed surgical and hospital treatment.

3 *A 54-year-old woman* was involved in a head-on accident in which she was wearing a seat belt. After the accident she complained of abdominal pain. It was found that she had facial injuries, a broken nose, a broken jaw on both sides, a ruptured spleen and ruptures of the intestines and small bowel. She developed numerous complications after surgery, such as blood clots in the lungs and other complications. She died of severe pneumonia in both lungs three weeks after admission to the hospital.

The types of injury reported above are typical of those caused by severe accidents when persons are wearing seat belts. The intestine appears to be cut apart by a shearing action between the external force of the impact and the spine. Blowout ruptures of the intestines are apparently caused by the sudden increase in pressure within a segment of the intestine within a closed loop as it is pressed against the vertebrae.

One thing should be emphasized about this kind of injury. It is an acceptable medical substitute for what might have occurred if the victim had not been wearing a seat belt. The magnitude of the problem, however, is revealed in another study that showed of 3,325 accident victims wearing seat belts, 944 were injured. Spinal injuries, pelvic fractures and injuries inside the abdomen were leading kinds of injuries apparently related to the wearing of a seat belt. However, just as many abdominal injuries occurred in persons not wearing seat belts. All physicians should carefully watch any seat belt victim who complains of abdominal pain.

blunt injuries to the chest

Bassett, Joseph S., Robert D. Gibson and Robert F. Wilson, "Blunt Injuries to the Chest," Journal of Trauma, 8: 418-429 (No. 3), May 1968.

Three surgeons from the Wayne State University School of Medicine, Detroit, Michigan observe that *chest injuries have become an increasing problem* in society today. It is estimated that one person dies of a chest injury every 40 minutes and that *one-fourth of all deaths caused by motor-vehicle accidents are due to chest injuries.*

The three surgeons report their findings and experiences from the case *records of 783 patients* admitted to the Detroit Receiving Hospital with blunt injury to the chest. Automobile accidents accounted for about one-half of the patients and falls for another one-fourth. [From these and other data, it appears that it is of great importance to maintain a clear airway for the victim and to get him to a well-equipped hospital.—Ed.]

The average chest-injury patient has three broken ribs, although the range was from 1 to 16. Other injuries within the chest included air, blood and air, or blood in the space between the inner part of the chest wall and the lung tissue; bruising of the lung tissue, rupture of the diaphragm and injury to an artery. Twenty-six per cent of the victims with chest injuries had these complications in addition to broken ribs. With each additional fractured rib there was an increase of approximately 10 per cent in the incidence of some other intra-chest injury.

Injuries outside the chest area were found to have *occurred in 25 per cent of the patients.* Fractures of the pelvis and/or spine, head injury, and a rupture of the liver, spleen, or other abdominal organ were most common. Fractures of the extremities were also common.

Forty-two patients reached the emergency room in shock and 50 per cent of them died. It was found that 71 per cent of the patients in shock had ruptured one of the large interior organs of the abdomen. The rupture of such organs was found to increase as the number of broken ribs increased. Thus, any victim of a chest injury with broken ribs must be suspected of having serious abdominal injuries as well.

Complications developed in 130 of the patients (17 per cent) and of this number *124 involved the respiratory system and/or pneumonia.* Thus, the major kinds of complications involving blunt injuries to the chest are apt, naturally enough, to involve the lungs, with pneumonia always a dominant complication.

Of the 56 deaths that occurred from chest injuries, 14 occurred from pneumonia or respiratory failure, 11 from heart failure; nine from hemorrhage, nine from associated head injuries, three from bleeding from the kidneys or bladder, two from blood clots to the lungs, two from septicemia (blood poisoning), two from kidney failure and four causes of death were undetermined.

The final outcome of any injury to the body depends upon the severity and frequency of associated injuries. Damage to the central nervous system and shock from hemorrhage are most dangerous. The so-called "wet-lung" which develops hours or days after the original chest injury because of inadequate removal of secretions is most serious; treatment is difficult and the final outcome is uncertain.

abdominal injuries

Hill, R. M. "Abdominal Injuries," The Practitioner, 192: 766-73, (No. 1152), June 1964.

A surgeon of the Cumberland Infirmary of Carlisle, England says that in considering abdominal injuries it should be remembered that *the spleen, especially when previously diseased, may be damaged by minor injury and it may bleed within its capsule for hours or days.*

Local tissue changes or a rise in blood pressure may start a major hemorrhage. Rupture of an abdominal muscle (such as the rectus) may result, with local pain, tenderness, and a protrusion when the torn muscle is contracted.

Rupture of the diaphragm occurs most commonly in crush injuries, and is often associated with injury to the spleen. Diagnosis is difficult, although the hearing of intestinal sounds in the chest may indicate the invasion of abdominal viscera through the ruptured diaphragm.

The liver is vulnerable to penetration and crush injuries. It is involved more often than suspected, although many liver injuries recover spontaneously. *The bile ducts are rarely injured,* although the presence of bile under the diaphragm indicates damage to these structures. Gross *injury to the pancreas* is serious, but rare. *The stomach is rarely injured,* but the duodenum may occasionally suffer direct violence or bursting by compression as the result of a fall on a hard object. Leakage of the contents is especially irritating in the presence of infection or injured tissues. *The small intestine* is often contused, but rupture is less common and probably results from the bursting of a compressed loop. Local spasm of the intestine that has ruptured may delay the emptying of contents into the abdominal cavity. Diagnosis of the injury may be delayed until peritonitis and general deterioration are evident. *The colon* is sometimes injured by gunshot and is less apt to be ruptured by crush or compression. *The rectum* may be torn or penetrated by a foreign body, enema nozzles and such. *The kidney* is involved in about 10 per cent of abdominal injuries. The cause is usually direct violence. Rupture produces pain in the loin, tenderness, and blood in the urine. *The bladder is less often injured* than the kidneys. Rupture of the bladder is usually by direct impact when it is full and injury is often associated with fracture of the pelvis. *The aorta* rarely ruptures in the abdomen. It is usually due to high-speed automobile accidents when it occurs.

Open injuries usually result from direct violence by impact or penetration and their significance is in proportion to the degree of involvement of internal organs. Closed injuries are more difficult to diagnose and accurate assessment may not be possible until the patient has recovered from shock and time has permitted signs of the injury to become evident. *A person suspected of an abdominal injury should be hospitalized.*

rupture of the spleen

Phillips, Charles A. Speas. *"Rupture of the Spleen," North Carolina Medical Journal, 18: 235-38 (No. 6), June 1957.*

Charles A. Speas Phillips, of Pinehurst, North Carolina, reports a study of 16 cases of rupture of the spleen.

In most cases the rupture of a spleen has been caused by an injury. Rupture of this organ may be frequently delayed, however, for some time after the initial injury.

A history of injury followed by dizziness, fainting, abdominal pain most severe in the left upper part of the abdomen and occasionally radiating to the left shoulder, abdominal tenderness and rigidity, increased pulse, shock, anemia, and other signs are associated with rupture of the spleen.

Accurate diagnosis, prompt treatment of shock, and surgical operation are necessary in the treatment of this emergency.

injury to the kidney

Casey, Murray Joseph. *"Renal Trauma," Military Medicine, 129: 136-142, (No. 2), February 1964.*

The staff physician of the U.S. Public Health Service Hospital in Boston observes that the highest incidence of kidney injuries occurs in active young males.

The most common causes of injury to the kidney today are direct blows, crushing, and indirect blows. Falls of even a short distance result in a sudden deceleration of the body, *while the kidney continues its downward course* and at times may be torn from its position. Although the kidney is an organ covered by a thin but strong capsule, it is surrounded by fatty tissue and fibrous tissue (fascia), so that "floating freely in its fat bed" it is subject to subtle injury.

Previous injury to the kidney, such as inflammation, stones, abscess, cysts, and other disorders, make the kidney more vulnerable to injury. Previous kidney disease is especially apt to be associated with kidney injuries in children.

The kidney may be injured in a variety of ways. It may be torn or lacerated, it may be partially or wholly separated from its pedicle (stalk), it may be bruised with internal hemorrhage and swelling, it may be lacerated or torn inside without damage to the covering capsule, it may be shattered into parts, or it may be damaged by the penetration of some object, such as a rib, a knife, or other object.

Bruises and contusions tend to heal in about four weeks, but if there is tearing or laceration through the capsule fibrous tissue will form over a longer period of time unless the kidney is repaired surgically.

Injuries to the kidney may be complicated by infections. The death of fragments of kidney tissue especially permit the growth of bacteria. Infections of the kidney can flare up quickly into serious disease of the kidney and may lead to its complete destruction or to distortion with the formation of scar tissue.

Signs and symptoms of kidney damage are multiple. The leading sign of injury to the kidney is blood in the urine, although blood may be seen only briefly. Pain in the flank or low back, with pain or tenderness in the abdomen, is present in from 60 to 80 per cent of kidney injuries. A mass in the flank (below the ribs of the back and above the pelvic bones) can be felt by the physician in about 20 per cent of the cases. Shock, with falling blood pressure and a fast pulse, may be present, and especially so if the kidney has been injured by penetration.

12
burns

Medical research on burns continues to occupy an important place in the practice of medicine. Both their prevention and their treatment represent partially unsolved challenges, although progress is being made along both lines. For the first aider the cold treatment of burn injuries represents a significant step forward in the last decade, both in the quick relief of pain and the ultimate achievement of better medical results.

Basic research has shown also that if the lungs can be protected against the inhalation of fire or smoke that injured persons may survive burns that would otherwise be fatal. Burns of children continue to provide a particular challenge to prevention, immediate first aid, and better medical care.

burns of children

Smith, E. Ide. "The Epidemiology of Burns," Pediatrics, 44: 821-27, (No. 5, Part II), November 1969.

A physician from the University of Oklahoma School of Medicine reports on *168 children admitted to a hospital* in Kansas City, Missouri *with acute burns* during the two-year period between January 1, 1966 and December 31, 1967.

Of the total of 168 patients, 95 were boys and 73 girls. *Thirteen of the patients had significant physical or emotional problems,* such as mental retardation (4), epilepsy (5), and organic brain disorder (2). One child was probably the victim of "abused child syndrome" who had multiple cigarette burns over her body. Three other children were intentionally burned by others.

The largest number of injuries, 124 of the 168, occurred as the result of the child's own actions. Only 37 children were innocent bystanders when injured. There were five deaths, or three per cent of the total. Four of the five deaths occurred from flame burns of more than fifty per cent of the total body surface.

The majority of burns were scalds, and the greatest number were seen *between the ages of 13 and 24 months.* The total number of burns appeared higher in the cold months. Most burns occurred at home, and most often in the kitchen.

No single factor was found to exist in every accident situation. There were, however, a number of factors which appeared to affect accident occurrence, such as disease problems of the child, chronic and acute stressful family situations, and accident repeatedness among family members.

Three areas of efforts at prevention are suggested:

(1) Flame-retardant fabric should be required by law. Two of five deaths in this group occurred from nightgown-type-burn injury.

(2) Appliances of improved design could minimize the possibilities of overturning and spilling.

(3) Open-flame heating units should carry a visual warning against the use of volatile liquids in proximity to the open flame. Several of the most serious flame burns and two deaths in this group resulted from this combination.

burning clothes

Oglesbay, Floyd B. "The Flammable Fabrics Problem," Pediatrics, 44: 827-32, (No. 5, Part II), November 1969.

Floyd B. Oglesbay, of the Injury Control Program, United States Public Health Service, Cincinnati, Ohio, points out that an estimated *3,000 deaths and 150,000 injuries occur annually in the United States from burns involving the ignition of clothing.*

Various studies indicate that *40 to 66 per cent of all burn cases involve the ignition of clothing.* One investigator assigned an "avoidability rating" for various types of burns. The preventability of clothing and flame burns ranked highest. In fact, the severity of clothing burns was nearly double that of the next type of burn, involving hot substances.

Medical treatment for severe burns is complex, time-consuming, and exceedingly expensive. Frequent operations and skin grafts are usually necessary. The mental anguish and stress are very serious; burn disfigurement often brings on feelings of guilt, insecurity, loneliness, and inferiority.

In considering fabrics as safe or unsafe, many factors must be considered. *Cotton and rayon generally burn the fastest. Synthetic fibers possess a somewhat lower potential for injury.* Fabrics made of animal hair, pure silk, and wool are the least hazardous. Napped surfaces usually burn quickly. In general, the heavier the fabric the higher its flame resistance. Long, loose-fitting garments are more dangerous than closer fitting clothes.

The Flammable Fabrics Act of 1954 set up national standards for testing and rating the flammability of clothing. *In 1967 an amendment* was signed by President Johnson to include all articles of wearing apparel and interior furnishings.

The future for less flammable fabrics is promising because American chemical and textile technology has made possible the use of *durable flame-retardant fibers* and fabrics. These fabrics are either inherently flame retardant or are made less flammable by the application of chemicals. Currently a number of such techniques are available, and many others are now being tested in the laboratory.

cold treatment of burns

Jung, Omero and Franklin V. Wade, "The Treatment of Burns with Ice Water, Phisohex, and Partial Hypothermia," Industrial Medicine and Surgery, 32: 365-70, (No. 9), September 1963.

Two surgeons of Hurley Hospital in Flint, Michigan report that the use of cold water in the first-aid treatment of burns and scalds is not new, since it has long been used by Icelanders.

Forty-six patients who were hospitalized for serious burns were treated by the two surgeons with ice water, Phisohex (germ-killing soap solution) and partial hypothermia (reduction of body temperature). Twenty-eight of the burned patients were ten years of age or younger. The burned area of the body was put immediately into a large basin containing water, ice, and Phisohex for from 45 minutes to 2 hours. If the body part could not be immersed in the ice water, cold wet towels or gauze squares kept in an ice bucket were applied to the burned area and changed frequently. Fresh ice was added as needed to keep the solution cold. Continuous cold compresses were applied in the hospital for 12 to 24 hours or even longer in some cases. If the burn was clean but extensive, it was covered with sterile towels in a normal salt solution and ice bags applied for at least 24 hours.

There was striking and immediate relief of pain on application of cold water to the burned part. Both pain and burning stopped immediately. The relief of pain was remarkedly better than with morphine or other pain-killing drugs. On treatment with cold, the red and infected areas did not develop blisters; the amount of swelling and loss of fluid was remarkedly decreased provided the cold was kept on for 24 hours. The rate of infection was low and the need for skin grafts was reduced, especially in second-degree burns.

When a burn occurs, not all the damage occurs at once. A great number of cells are injured rather than killed by the burn. These injured cells permit the loss of fluid and many cells die. The final result is an external loss of water, electrolytes (minerals) and proteins. Cold appears to slow down this whole process by constricting the blood vessels, decreasing capillary permeability, and reducing the oxygen demand of the cell, with a resultant drop in cellular metabolism.

In this study of burn injuries the ice water treatment was judged to be a superior method of treatment because it: 1) gave immediate pain relief; 2) decreased swelling and loss of fluid, protein, and electrolytes; 3) prevented infection and 4) gave better healing results.

burns on the face

Phillips, Anne Wight, and Oliver Cope. "Burn Therapy — III. Beware the Facial Burn!" Annals of Surgery, 156: 759-66, (No. 5), November 1962.

Two physicians of the Department of Surgery, Harvard Medical School report that *injuries to the lungs and respiratory tract* in general *are a principal killer of the burned patient. A study of 398 burned patients* revealed that most of the injury to the lungs occurs when the flames are in an enclosed space.

Evidence of burns to the face represent an important clue to possible respiratory damage. In this study 46 per cent of the patients who had burns of the face died from injuries to the lungs, in contrast to 11 per cent who died from flame burns without injuries to the face.

The following *major conclusions were made from this study:*

1 *Respiratory (lung) damage should be suspected in every patient with deep flame burns around the nose and mouth.* Approximately nine out of ten burned patients with facial damage will have lung damage.

2 *The risk of death is much greater for persons with second and third degree burns of the mouth and nose.* Persons with equally extensive burns whose faces escape injury tend to be spared (they have escaped lung damage).

3 *There is not such risk of death if the face is burned elsewhere* than around the nose and mouth.

4 *Respiratory tract damage may occur in people who have been overcome by smoke, even though there is no facial burn.*

5 The majority of patients with flame burns of more than 40 per cent of the body surface will also have second or third degree burns of the respiratory tract.

6 Confinement of both patient and fire in *an enclosed space increases the probability that the lungs will be damaged* by flame and heat, or smoke.

7 Deep flame burns of the respiratory tract that have occurred out-of-doors do not cause as much respiratory difficulty as injury from an enclosed space.

8 *Flame burns are more deadly than liquid burns, due to respiratory damage.*

9 *Longer hospitalization is* required for the patient with facial burns.

critical results of burns

Phillips, Anne Wight, and Oliver Cope. "Burn Therapy - II. The Revelation of Respiratory Tract Damage as a Principal Killer of the Burned Patient," Annals of Surgery, 155: 1-19, (No. 1), January 1962.

Two physicians of the Department of Surgery of the Harvard Medical School examined the medical records of 106 persons who had died from burns at the Massachusetts General Hospital over a period of 18 years. The following major conclusions regarding death from burns were reached from this investigation:

1 *The prime killer of the burned patient is respiratory damage.* In this study, 42 per cent of the deaths occurred from this cause.

2 Infection of the damaged respiratory tract becomes apparent as a rule if the patient survives for 72 hours. Isolation helps.

3 Shock, which accounted for 20 per cent of all deaths through the year 1947, has now become an insignificant factor in burns. Only one person died from shock due to burns over a ten-year period. The reduction in deaths from shock represents improvement in the medical methods of treating shock.

4 *Damage to the kidneys and death from uremia have increased* as the patient is able to survive longer than in previous years. Approximately nine per cent of the burned patients in this study died from uremia after eight or more days of survival.

5 Pulmonary emboli (clots or obstructions of the blood vessels in the lungs) accounted for three per cent of the burn deaths in this study. The emboli in the lungs caused three deaths and there were clots or obstructions (emboli) in the lungs of at least seven more burned patients, although they were not judged to be a cause of death.

6 Cardiac disease caused the death of eight patients in this group of burned patients. However, all eight of the deaths occurred in persons who had pre-existing heart disease.

7 *Miscellaneous causes of deaths* were observed in a minority of cases. Massive hemorrhage in the adrenal glands, pre-existing illness such as brain tumor, brain hemorrhage, liver disease and other causes were involved in isolated cases.

There is mounting evidence that in a conflagration the danger of respiratory damage can be diminished by covering the face with a wet cloth.

biologic treatment of burns

Bromberg, Bertram E. "Burn Wound Management with Biologic Dressings," New York State Journal of Medicine, 70: 1645-1646, (No. 12), June 15, 1970.

The medical director of plastic surgery at Kings County Medical Center in Brooklyn, New York reports that *biologic dressings have proved to be of great value in the treatment of serious burn wounds. Biologic dressings are applied over burns only for a temporary period of time.* Biologic dressings are from human or animal tissues, applied in plastic surgery to the burned surface. Despite living donors, cadavers, and tissue banks there is a shortage of biologic materials for burns.

The homograft involves the use of tissues from the body of another of the same species. Thus, a graft from another human would be a homograft. The rejection phenomenon is applicable to skin grafts from another person just as it is in heart transplants or other organ transplants, but for the treatment of burns the skin graft from another person (homograft) is applied only temporarily and is removed before the material can be rejected. In the meantime the firm adherence of the graft has prevented the loss of protein, electrolytes (electrically charged minerals) and body heat and has diminished pain and the production of fibroblasts (which would cause scarring). It also prevents much infection and permits a less-painful dressing change. When applied over joint surfaces the graft may permit painless motion and minimize contractures. If removal is done before the rejection phenomenon it is less painful because adherence is less firm and less bleeding is encountered. The process is continued with a new homograft until an autograft from the patient himself can be performed.

The xenograft involves the use of tissue from other animals than the human, such as the pig. Dog xenografts have been employed successfully and so have embryo skins from cattle. Pig skin is usually devoid of any local reactions and does not show adverse responses.

Although many synthetic products have been developed they are not satisfactory because they have no capacity for resisting bacteria such as homografts and xenografts possess.

Dr. Bromberg says there is no doubt that temporary biologic dressings have become a part of burn wound management. Homografts and pig xenografts are the best covering agents at present. Both, however, are temporary and must be replaced.

13
electrical injuries

Electrical injuries are apt to be far more extensive in their nature than a source of burns alone. Electrical burns of the mouth, usually involving children, are apt to be difficult for the physician or surgeon because of tissue destruction that may go unrecognized. Neurological and psychological results of electrical injuries in surviving victims may be extensive and long lasting, depending upon severity of the former and personalities of the latter.

The first aider must be aware of his first responsibility following separation of the victim from the source of current—namely, the administration of emergency measures to support life. However, he must also know some of the diagnostic difficulties and later complications of electrical injuries so that he can assist the physician in giving further care.

electrical burns of the mouth

Blandford, Sidney E. *"Electrical Burns of the Mouth in Children," Rocky Mountain Medical Journal*, 65: 25-28 (No. 6), June, 1968.

A physician of Denver, Colorado observes that *electrical burns of the mouth* occur mostly in small children between the ages of one and two years.

Multiple-outlet extension cords lying on the floor at home with at least one of the usual three outlets open are involved in most of the electrical injuries of the mouth in these small children. The child sucks the open outlet, *the saliva completes the circuit* and an electrical burn of the mouth occurs.

Chewing a light cord is a rare cause of an electrical burn in a child. Usually it is the saliva in a child's mouth that is involved in an electrical injury of this kind. It is through the saliva that the circuit is completed.

Electrical burns of the mouth in children are disfiguring. Healing is slow and disfigurement of the mouth is apt to occur despite all efforts at reconstruction. Reconstruction of the mouth and associated tissues by the plastic surgeon should be deferred for a year or more until the blood supply to the affected tissues has recovered, scars have softened and as much tissue as possible has been salvaged.

Over a period of 13 years at the Denver Hospital there were 87 admissions for electrical burns of the mouth. However, these admissions represented only *44 different patients.*

When a child puts an electrical outlet in the mouth the saliva conducts the electricity and the moist mucous membrane of the mouth offers little resistance to the passage of electricity. The tip of the tongue is often involved in the contact with electrical current. Theoretically, if the child had wet diapers and was sitting on a hot air register that was grounded through the furnace, the contact from the "hot side" could ground itself and result in death of the child.

Electrical burns of the mouth in children can be prevented in the following ways: 1) restrictions in the use of electrical extension cords; 2) the use of "self-closing outlets" or safety caps for the wall outlets; 3) the use of electrical cords with self-closing outlets or only a single opening; 4) taping of multiple outlet cords to cover unused openings. Although most packaged safety devices for the prevention of electrical burns of the mouth emphasize the putting of metal objects in the outlets by children, none mention sucking at the outlet which is the more common cause of electrical burns of the mouth.

electrical injuries

Sturim, Howard S. "Electrical Burns: Good Functional and Cosmetic Result Related to Choice of Early Excision or Conservative Therapy," Rhode Island Medical Journal, 51: 42-45 (No. 1), January 1968.

A member of the Department of Surgery of the Rhode Island Hospital in Providence says *the frequency of electrical burns is on the increase,* and these kinds of injuries must be better understood.

Electric *current of less than 1,000 volts is considered a low tension current.* Above this voltage the current is high tension. Such wires usually carry alternating current which is considered as approximately three times more dangerous than direct current of similar intensity. The alternations of current cause tetanic spasms which make the victim grip the wires or electrodes more firmly and increase the difficulty of detachment. *Domestic sixty cycle alternating current is very dangerous to the heart and the respiratory center.* The degree of tissue damage in an electric injury is proportional to the intensity of current which passes through the victim.

The *resistance of various body tissues* to the flow of an electrical current decreases in magnitiude in the following order: bone, fat, tendon, skin, muscle, blood and nerve. After an electric current has penetrated the skin, it passes rapidly through the tissue fluids and along blood vessels. However, there are many factors that determine individual susceptibility. For example, the resistance offered by the calloused palm may reach 1,000,000 ohms, while the average normal skin resistance is about 5,000 ohms. The moist skin may offer as little resistance as 1,000 ohms.

In electrical burns *the tissues may be heated momentarily to temperatures of 2,500 degrees Centigrade to 3,000 degrees Centigrade.* The heat is proportional to the square of the current flow. In the body the current flows along the paths of least resistance. The current is most concentrated at the points of entrance or exit and it is at these points that coagulation of tissue may occur.

Once the flow of current through the victim takes place, the path of the flow determines death or survival. Currents that pass through the heart or brain stem may cause immediate death. Unconsciousness and convulsions indicate early central nervous system injury. Permanent damage to the brain or spinal cord may occur in survivors. Fractures and dislocations may occur also because of severe muscle contractions due to electrical stimulation. Electrical injuries involving the head may cause cataracts of the eyes. Late complications such as severe hemorrhage, progressive deficiency of blood in body parts, and gangrene may occur because of the destruction of blood vessels. Blood clots may occur.

Separation of the victim from electrical contact is the first step in an electrical accident. Immediate *artificial respiration* and *cardiac massage* will save many victims of electrical shock. *In the hospital,* or under the care of a physician, the use of oxygen, intravenous fluids, antibiotics, tetanus immunization and local wound hygiene may help the patient recover.

Burns of the mouth are frequent in children. Such electrical burns involve the mouth, lips, and tongue. Loss of the incisors may occur, so that damage to teeth should always be investigated. The scars that form after electrical injuries to the mouth of children may cause severe deformities from contraction as the wound heals, if no reconstructive, plastic efforts are employed. Thus, the plastic surgeon should be consulted in electrical injuries to the mouth of children. If the corner of the mouth is destroyed by electrical burn, then the upper and lower lips adhere and the size of the mouth is reduced.

Electrical burns of the hand have created much controversy among physicians. This part of the body is injured more frequently by electrical burns than other parts and too often there is excessive scar tissue formation, contracture of the fingers and stiffness of the joints that result in limited function of the hand.

Although infections associated with electrical burns are not considered to be of great significance, gas gangrene can occur and overwhelming infections with other bacteria have been documented as a cause of death in electrical burn victims; thus the physician must control infections if possible.

The depth of an electrical burn cannot be estimated easily soon after the injury. Often many weeks will pass after the injury before the doctor can accurately judge the amount of damage that has been done.

electrical accidents

Kouwenhoven, W. B., "Electricity and the Human Body," National Safety News, 63:30 ff., (No. 2), February 1951.

W. B. Kouwenhoven reports that the passage of an electric current through the body produces numerous effects that differ in intensity and kind. They range all the way from a slight tingling sensation to death. The effects may be good or bad. In certain mental diseases an electric shock may have a healing influence, or it may produce either a state of depression, characterized by rapid, weak pulse, shallow breathing, pallor, restlessness, and a depressed mental state similar to surgical shock, or a highly excited state. The effects of electrical shock may be classified as follows:

1 *Conscious phenomena.* If the victim of an electric shock retains consciousness, there is often a ringing or whistling in the ears and there may be partial deafness for a time. In addition, some visual disorders involving flashes and brilliant spots of colors may occur. Pain and soreness in the muscles are common. The victim is often restless and irritable. These symptoms usually subside after a few hours.

2 *Muscle contractions.* A contraction of muscles takes place when contact is made with an electric circuit. The severity of this muscle contraction accounts for the soreness of muscles that is felt after electrical shock.

3 *Convulsions.* Convulsions may take place; they are usually of an irregular muscle-spasm type with tremors.

4 *Electric-shock treatment.* Electric shock is used by psychiatrists in the treatment of certain types of mental illness. It is most effective in the treatment of depression. These treatments usually result in a marked impairment of memory, and memory usually returns completely a few weeks after the treatment is stopped. Marked changes are recorded in the brain waves.

5 *Narcosis.* When an electric current, passing through the brain of a patient, produces convulsions, there follows a period of unconsciousness lasting several minutes. Some doctors have attempted to produce periods of narcosis but without convulsions by using lower current.

6 *Electric burns.* The true electric burn is often characterized by a pinkish or reddish spot on the burned area at the surface of the skin. Such burns, however, may penetrate deeply and require considerable time to heal. Burns, blisters, and markings are not necessarily present on the skin after an electrical accident. When the skin is saturated with water and the contact area is large, a fatal shock may not leave the slightest detectable blemish. Burns produced by electricity usually heal slowly and without infection.

7 *Loss of consciousness.* A victim of electric shock may lose consciousness. In some instances, he may recover spontaneously; in others, only after the application of artificial respiration.

8 *Emission.* Ejaculation of seminal fluid is common in males and occurs at low as well as at high voltages. The severe muscular contraction is believed to be responsible for this phenomenon.

9 *Incontinence.* The victims of electric shock are in some cases incontinent for a while, and sometimes blood is present in the urine.

10 *Rise in blood pressure.* An electric shock that does not stop the heart is usually followed by a rise in blood pressure. The pressure usually remains high for a period, gradually returning to normal.

11 *Hemorrhages.* Small hemorrhages are sometimes found in the brain, the spinal cord, and other organs. The eyes may be bloodshot because of the rupturing of blood vessels.

12 *The nervous system.* Contact with electric circuit may cause profound shock, or so fatigue the nervous system that it will not function normally for a period of minutes or hours. One of the most common effects is temporary paralysis.

13 *Permanent effects.* Permanent damage to nerves by paralysis following electric shock is extemely rare, but it sometimes occurs. Usually, pain and weakness follow the accident. Most victims either die immediately or recover, although perhaps only after extensive burns have healed.

14 *Death.* Death from electric shock may result from a single cause or from a combination of two or more factors, In general, low voltages and small current shocks kill through action on the heart, and high voltages kill through either the destruction or the inhibition of nerve centers, with asphyxia, or cessation of breathing, as the common, immediate cause of death.

deaths from lightning

Metropolitan Life Insurance Company. "The Death Toll from Lightning." Statistical Bulletin 28 7-9, (No. 6), June 1947.

Lightning kills around 400 persons annually in the United States, or about three in every million of the population. The probability of being fatally injured by lightning is far greater in rural than in urban areas.

City dwellers are relatively safe, one reason being that the steel structures of the tall buildings act as lightning conductors. Moreover, persons in urban areas, when caught in a sudden thunderstorm, usually do not have far to go to reach a place of shelter. Rural dwellers, on the other hand, are more likely to be caught some distance from a safe shelter, and to find themselves a target for the electric discharge, particularly when they are on a broad plain.

Many lives are lost each year because of the dangerous actions of persons caught in thunderstorms. This is evident from a study of the death claim records of persons insured in the Industrial Department of the Metropolitan Life Insurance Company who had been killed by lightning during the years 1941-45. *One-third of the victims lost their lives when they sought shelter under a tree; by so doing they increased the danger of being struck.* Trees, and particularly isolated trees, because of their height, are more likely to be struck than persons; and after striking the tree, the bolt may flash sideways or, after reaching the base of the tree, it may run along the ground and strike anyone in its path. Ironically enough, a number of those killed among the insured were standing under trees only a short distance from their homes. *Homes properly equipped with lightning rods afford virtually complete safety. Similarly, the metal bodies of automobiles protect the occupants, even if the vehicle is struck by lightning.*

The practice of seeking refuge in small sheds, especially in exposed areas, is also dangerous. These structures are a more likely target than are individuals.

Persons in small boats, it should be realized, are conspicuous targets, while swimmers are in danger not only of being struck directly, but also of being electrocuted by a charge carried by the water from a bolt striking some distance away.

14
heat injuries

Serious injury of a permanent nature may occur to many organs of the body when a person survives damage from high temperatures. Clinical experience and research of physicians have shown that exercise in hot weather may cause deaths or internal injuries of a most serious nature in some persons, even though they are young and in good physical condition.

Rapid cooling, preferably with the use of ice or icewater baths, represents the most effective first aid for persons suffering heat injuries of a serious nature.

fatalities and medical effects of heat and exercise

Schrier, Robert W., Haller S. Henderson, C. Craig Tisher and Richard L. Tannen. "Nephropathy Associated with Heat Stress and Exercise," Annals of Internal Medicine, 67: 356-376 (No. 2), August 1967.

Four army physicians of the Department of Metabolism, Division of Medicine, Walter Reed Army Institute of Research in Washington, D.C. report eight cases in which army recruits between the ages of 19 and 24 years suffered severe kidney damage from heatstroke that occurred during military activities of a physical nature during hot weather. Five of the victims died.

Autopsy studies of the kidneys showed them to be enlarged (swollen) and to have abnormalities or death of individual cells of the kidneys. Damage to the kidneys was considered by the physicians to be due to dehydration (loss of body fluid), collapse of the circulatory system. high body temperature and the actions of pigments and hemoglobin from the destruction of blood cells.

During the hospital treatment of the heatstroke victims much destructive metabolism (breakdown of living cells) was observed to be occurring, there was damage to the muscles, persistent fevers without evidence of infections, widespread involvement of different systems of the body and prolonged periods of time when the patients could not urinate. In three fatal cases extensive degeneration of muscle tissue was found to have occurred.

Complications involving the central nervous system (brain and spinal cord), the blood forming system, the liver, the heart and circulatory system and gastrointestinal tract made treatment of the kidney failure more difficult.

Lung congestion and swelling (edema), hemorrhage into the heart, destruction of liver cells, excessive amounts of blood in the brain and degeneration of skeletal muscles was frequently found on autopsy in the patients who died from the heatstroke that developed during exercise in hot weather.

Symptoms, clinical observations, laboratory tests, and autopsy findings on these eight victims of heatstroke indicate that *physical activity of a vigorous nature during excessively hot weather may produce profound and extensive body changes that may result in death or extended illness.*

Treatment for the heatstroke victims involved the *use of ice water baths, vigorous cooling with ice packs,* intravenous fluids, tranquilizing agents, and a variety of technical hospital procedures to support kidney and other functions.

Illnesses associated with heat stress have worldwide importance, but according to these physicians, the problem has received little attention in the United States.

four effects of excessive heat

Ross, Frank. "Medical Problems Related to the Hostile Environment; III. Problems Related to Heat," Southwestern Medicine, 47: 137-42, (No. 5), May 1966.

Captain Frank Ross, MC, points out that *the human body loses heat primarily through the skin.* Disorders of heat regulation are usually caused by: (1) severe environmental *temperature greater than body temperature;* (2) moderate environmental *temperature with high humidity,* or (3) *lack of circulation of surrounding air.*

The disorders of heat regulation discussed below are probably a spectrum of one basic disorder in which the heat-regulatory mechanism is respectively more severely deranged and thus the symptoms more disturbing.

1 *Heat cramps.* Symptoms are *severe spasms in the legs and abdomen.* Primarily affected are workers performing a great deal of physical exercise in a warm, humid climate. The basic difficulty is inadequate salt replacement after excessive sweating. The condition is not serious and can be prevented by adding salt to drinking water.

2 *Heat exhaustion.* This condition is characterized by *profuse sweating, cool, clammy skin, weak pulse, headache, dizziness, confusion, nausea, and visual disturbances.* Treatment consists of removal to a cool, well-aerated area, and administering fluids (preferably with salt). The prognosis is good and recovery complete.

3 *Heat exhaustion without perspiration.* The symptoms are similar to heat exhaustion, except that there is no perspiration: *the skin is dry.* Body temperature may be elevated. This condition usually occurs when humidity is very high. Treatment is the same as for heat exhaustion.

4 *Heatstroke.* Unlike the previous conditions, *heatstroke is very serious and is a medical emergency.* It occurs *chiefly in the elderly, the obese, during acute alcoholic states, and in people with chronic diseases. Almost all people suffering heatstroke will die if not treated. In heatstroke, the person suddenly ceases to sweat and body temperature rises rapidly.* Headache, confusion, staggering gait, delirium, and finally, coma, usually with convulsions, develop. The skin is hot, red, and dry. Pulse is rapid. The *best treatment is immediate immersion in an ice water bath until body temperature is less than 102˚*. If the victim recovers, there may be residual damage to the central nervous system, heart, liver, and kidneys. There is greater liability to subsequent heatstroke attacks. Prevention of this disorder is vital. *In heat, short periods of exposure, frequent rest, adequate fluids, and proper clothing are important.*

heat stroke

Baxter, Charles R., and Paul E. Teschan, "Atypical Heat Stroke, with Hypernatremia, Acute Renal Failure, and Fulminating Potassium Intoxication," Archives of Internal Medicine, 101: 1040-50, (No. 6), June, 1958.

Two physicians of the United States Army Medical Corps from Fort Sam Houston, Texas observe that the criteria for the diagnosis of heat stroke are well known, but abnormal behavior without severe elevation of body temperature may go unrecognized as heatstroke, even though the disorder is ultimately identified. Heat stroke sometimes is mistaken for an acute mental disorder.

Two vital principles in the treatment of heat stroke are the *rapid lowering of the body temperature and the rapid restoration of the blood volume.* In heat stroke there is a great increase in vascular space, due to the dilation of blood vessels. In effect, this enlargement of space has the effect of reducing the blood volume. Rapid administration of salt and water may be needed to meet the discrepancy between the existing blood volume and the expanded vascular space. With rapid cooling there is less need for body fluids.

Rapid lowering of body temperature is best accomplished in severe cases by immersion in ice water until the temperature falls below 101 degrees F. Alcohol sponging may be effective when high fever and shock are not present. This can be accomplished when two people rub vigorously with iced alcohol sponges in an adequate draft.

In this study three patients died from heatstroke. It was thought that death was due to the following factors:

(1) Destruction of body cells because of the prolonged high fever and severe lack of oxygen due to shock conditions.

(2) Elevation of the sodium content of the blood due to the loss of body fluid from sweating and the giving of sodium chloride (salt). It was thought that the mental disorder symptoms of the three patients were due to the high sodium content of the blood.

(3) Destruction of heat-damaged red blood cells.

(4) Movement of potassium out of the cells into the blood with rapid development of potassium intoxication.

salt losses in hot environments

Weiner, J. S., and R. E. van Heyninggen. "Salt Losses of Men Working in Hot Environments," *British Journal of Industrial Medicine, 9: 56-64, (No. 1), January 1952.*

J. S. Weiner and R. E. van Heyninggen of the Medical Research Council Climate and Working Efficiency Research Unit at Oxford, England, report that the necessity for an adequate salt intake for people working in hot climates has been recognized for a long time. Salt deficiency is known to cause heat cramps and lesser degrees of ill-health and efficiency.

This study was concerned with the measurement of sweat and urinary loss of salt under working conditions in a hot environment. *It was found that there is substantial loss of body salt in a hot climate and that this deficiency should be replaced.*

Under conditions where men sweat profusely at a water-output of about five quarts a day and over, there is probably a salt loss of about three grams per working hour. At this salt-loss level the daily requirement for replacement would be about twenty to twenty-four grams of salt. This figure is close to the average intake, as actually measured, of men working in tropical climates.

In most cases in a hot climate it is necessary to supplement the diet with about ten grams of salt.

265 cases of heat disease

Borden, Daniel L., James F. Waddill, and George S. Grier III. "Statistical Study of 265 Cases of Heat Disease," *Journal of the American Medical Association, 128: 1200-1205, (No. 17), August 25, 1945.*

Colonel Daniel L. Borden, Lieutenant Colonel James F. Waddill, and Captain George S. Grier III, of the Army Medical Corps, report a study of 265 cases of heat disease in troops training at Fort Eustis.

The effects of heat accumulation in the body are generally grouped under the term of heat disease and include the following:

1 *Heat cramps* (muscle cramps from salt loss). This is, however, not entirely specific for heat cases alone, as it may occur in any environment as a result of salt and fluid loss.

2 *Heat prostration,* characterized by weakness, usually some temperature elevation, loss of appetite, headache, abdominal distress, nausea, vomiting, and visual disturbances.

3 *Heat exhaustion,* when evidence of circulatory failure is present in addition to the effects of heat accumulation. High temperature may or may not be present, depending on the degree of shock present.

4 *Heat stroke,* representing a failure of the heat regulatory mechanisms, with fever as the predominant feature; coma may or may not be present.

The onset of heat distress may be gradual and insidious and elicit only casual attention, but an abrupt rapid change into one of the more serious forms is not uncommon.

The accompanying table shows the statistical data on the symptoms of heat disease based on observations of 265 cases.

Symptoms	Mild Cases (Percentage)	Severe Cases (Percentage)
Fever (over 99.6°F.)	78.0	100.0
Dyspnea (difficult breathing)	48.0	100.0
Tachycardia (fast heart)	40.0	100.0
Vertigo (dizziness)	74.0	88.0
Coma (unconsciousness)	0.0	84.0
Systolic blood pressure under 100 mm. of Hg.	4.0	75.0
Headache	19.0	53.0
Cyanosis	5.0	50.0
Anxiety-apprehension	31.0	37.0
Nausea	18.0	13.0
Muscle cramps	14.0	13.0
Vomiting	5.0	13.0
Spasm of feet and hands	8.0	0.0

Three fatalities occurred in men who had undergone strenuous physical exertion under adverse climatic conditions. One of these men was found to have died in his barracks during the night, following a day of strenuous physical activity. In all three deaths hemorrhages were common.

In several nonfatal cases with pronounced fever, scattered subcutaneous hemorrhages over the surface of the trunk and extremities were also noted.

The following conclusions were drawn from the study.

(1) In a climate with a high atmospheric temperature, high humidity, and a low wind-velocity the incidence of pathologic effect from heat on the human body tends to be high.

(2) The initial effects of heat accumulation in human beings may be

mild and of insidious onset, eliciting only casual attention in its early stages. Such a condition, however, may abruptly and rapidly change into one of the more severe stages of the disorder accompanied by a high fatality rate.

(3) Heat loss in man is chiefly accomplished by radiation, convection, conduction, and vaporization of water.

(4) As the external temperature rises about 30°C. (86°F.), vaporization of water becomes the increasingly predominant means of heat loss in the human body, until at or near 35°C. (95°F.) it is practically the sole means of heat dissipation.

(5) While vaporization of water from the skin surface depends mainly on the degree of saturation of the air with moisture (relative humidity), the wet bulb temperature seems a more sensitive indicator of the probable incidence of heat disease at high atmospheric temperatures than the relative humidity.

(6) Strenuous physical activity under adverse climatic conditions strongly increases the incidence of heat effects, especially when performed by persons not acclimatized.

(7) In the treatment of the more severe cases in which circulatory failure or shock is present or impending, the intravenous administration of one to two units of plasma is recommended over the use of saline solution, owing to the ready diffusibility of the latter into the tissues.

(8) The use of 100 per cent oxygen by mask has proved advantageous in the treatment of shock in heat disease.

It is apparent that extremely high temperatures may cause severe illness or death if proper precautions are not taken.

15
cold injuries

The importance of wind in conjunction with low temperatures has been established by research and medical experience in arctic areas. The speed with which freezing can occur has an almost amazing association with wind velocities and temperatures. Military experiences of the past 20 years or more have shown that frostbite and other cold injuries may have great significance in battle operations.

Both emergency and chronic effects of cold are being studied by medical investigators. Frostbite in a child, for example, may cause permanent damage to the growing part of the long bones, with ultimate reduction in height. The importance of rapid warming of frozen tissues continues to be a mainstay of first aid for persons saved from freezing.

effects of frostbite on growth

Lindholm, A., Olov Nilsson and F. Svartholm. "Epiphyseal Destruction Following Frostbite," Acta Chirurgica Scandinavica, 134: 37-40, (No. 1), 1968.

Three Swedish physicians report that *frostbite may cause serious damage to the epiphysis of a bone.* (The epiphysis, located at the end of a bone, is separated from the bone itself by cartilage that permits the bone to grow; thus, damage to the epiphysis may interfere with growth).

The Swedish physicians observe that *there is considerable information on the blood and circulatory effects of frostbite.* Inflammation, blood clots, swelling, hemorrhage and gangrene have all been reported as resulting from frostbite. Animal experiments have shown, however, that *certain cartilage cells are highly sensitive to cold* and that they may be damaged directly by the latter and not as a secondary complication due to changes in the blood and circulation. Some animal studies have shown that cartilage may be damaged within 30 minutes after refrigeration.

The first medical report on epiphyseal destruction in the fingers was reported in 1930, although additional reports have been made of such damage in young children since that date.

In this report the physicians describe *three cases of damage to the growth of the fingers* because of frostbite. In one case a 2-year-old boy was outside for 20 minutes in a temperature of 25 degrees below zero Centigrade without gloves on his hands. When his parents found him his hands and arms were swollen, white, and in a condition that a physician diagnosed within one hour as first-degree frostbite. The hands appeared to be normal by the next day, but 18 months later the growth of two fingers on each hand was abnormal due to epiphyseal damage.

In another case *a Lapp of four years of age was outside for 15 minutes at a temperature of 30 degrees below freezing Centigrade.* He was warmly dressed, but had *no gloves* and froze both hands. Although the hands appeared to heal well, the fingers were observed to be abnormal after about one year. The abnormality in growth of the fingers was judged to have resulted from cold injury to the growing part of the bones of the fingers.

The third case involved *a female child whose fingers froze fast to a bucket at the age of 2 years.* The father had to wrench the hands free. Blistering and loss of skin occurred from the frostbite, but recovery appeared until characteristic finger deformities appeared about one year later which were judged to be due to cold injury to the epiphyses.

X-ray studies confirmed the partial or complete destruction of the epiphyses of the involved bones. Shortening of the fingers and deviation or bending of the ends of the fingers occur because of early injury to the growing part of the bone. The thumbs were not involved.

accidental deaths from cold weather

Staff. "Accidental Hypothermia," *British Medical Journal*, 2: 1471, (No. 5528), December 17, 1966.

A study of 126 persons who were admitted to selected hospitals with low body temperatures from *exposure to cold* was conducted by a Committee of the Royal College of Physicians in Great Britain. The study has revealed certain significant relationships.

Most of the cold injuries occurred when the external temperature dropped below 41 degrees Fahrenheit. No age was immune from danger, but the very young and the very old were especially susceptible. Of the total number of patients *24 per cent were below the age of one year and 42 per cent were over the age of 65 years.*

The old people who suffered from cold exposure were usually those who lived alone and who were sleeping in poorly heated homes or outdoors. *The babies* had inadequate mothers or cold homes. One child fell into a freezing lake. Diseases were often present; mostly congenital defects (present at birth) in the babies and heart disease, diabetes, or some due to drugs in the old persons.

No patient survived if he had a body temperature below 80 degrees Fahrenheit when admitted to the hospital. Even if the body temperature was *between 93 to 95 degrees Fahrenheit (by rectal temperature) the death rate was 30 per cent.* Deaths for the total group of 126 patients amounted to *37 per cent* (47 deaths).

A Major Problem: On the basis of this study involving just a few hospitals, the Committee calculated that *for Great Britain as a whole about 9,000 persons are admitted to hospitals during the three months in winter because of accidental exposure to cold.* During the winter months exposure to *cold is one of the major causes of death in England.* Preventive measures should be taken seriously, especially to protect infants and old people.

The tradition that bedroom windows should be kept open needs to be overcome, say these authorities, and the importance of adequate heating in the home should be stressed. More food is needed in cold weather for a person to stay warm. Improvement in the insulation of some homes may be advisable. It should become more widely known that welfare officials will often make funds available for fuel with which to keep the house warm. Neighbors should visit old people who live alone during cold weather to check on their welfare. A thermometer should be kept in the home and any temperature below 41 degrees F. should be recognized as a hazard. Persons suffering from cold may not look ill. When a person feels cold to touch underneath his clothing his temperature should be taken by rectal thermometer for five minutes. If the body temperature is below 95 degrees F. the victim should be hospitalized for treatment and care should be taken to keep the victim warm while he is enroute to the hospital.

injury from excessive cold

Birk, Thomas C. "Medical Problems Related to the Hostile Environment; IV. Problems Related to Cold," Southwestern Medicine, 47: 142-43, (No. 5), May 1966.

Major Thomas C. Birk, MC, reports that *cold injuries have been of primary concern to the military forces* because of their importance in many campaigns, such as Napoleon's in Poland, and Hitler's in Russia. In World War II in the U. S. Army, there were a total of 90,535 time-lost injuries due to cold.

The type of injury produced is divided into four categories: *chilblains, immersion foot, trench foot, and frost bite. Chilblains* result from exposure to temperatures above freezing in high humidity and produce a painful redness of the skin which clears rapidly on warming. *Immersion foot* results from exposure for from 12 hours to seven days to water at temperatures usually below 50°. *Trench foot* results from prolonged exposure to cold and wetness at 20-50°. *Frostbite* is actual crystallization of tissue fluids in the skin, occurring after exposure of only a few seconds to several hours, at below freezing temperatures.

Cold is the main factor producing cold injuries, but this is enhanced by wind or moisture, which removes skin heat. Children and elderly people are the most susceptible, while in the military the lower ranks experience the most cold injuries.

Previous cold injuries, fatigue, training, discipline, nutrition, health, and psychosociological factors all play a role in producing cold injuries. *The Negro is approximately six times more vulnerable than the Caucasian*, and his injury is usually more severe.

Cold injuries often have an insidious onset with a tingling or mild aching sensation being the only symptoms, followed by numbness.

The treatment of cold injuries can be divided into emergency first aid treatment and subsequent hospital care. If the victim has to walk, thawing should be delayed. If he can be evacuated by litter, then *rapid thawing should be performed as soon as possible by placing the frostbitten extremity in a warm bath. The use of snow, rubbing of the extremity, various ointments, ingestion of alcohol, and tobacco is to be avoided.* The best treatment of cold injuries is prevention. Adequate, protective, dry, clean clothing of many layers is most useful. *Almost all cold injuries can be prevented* if proper precautions are taken.

the windchill factor

Cold, wind, and dampness are major threats to survival in an arctic temperature. Chills and shivering are the first danger signals to the possibility of injury or death by cold. *The Windchill Factor* is a number, evolved from research, that combines the effects of the speed of wind and the temperature of the environment. The stronger the wind or the lower the temperature the higher the windchill factor.

184 cold injuries

Windchill Factor	Effects
1200	Bitterly cold
1400	Exposed flesh may freeze
2000	Exposed flesh will freeze in less than one minute
2300	Exposed flesh freezes in less than *30 seconds*.

Example: If the temperature is minus 30 degrees F. and the wind is calm, a standing man will be very cold. If he starts to move then wind movement becomes a factor. If he walks at three miles per hour the exposed parts of his body will be subject to *frostbite*. If he rides in an open truck at 15 mph frostbite will develop almost immediately.

Frostbite is the freezing of living tissue. The first symptom is a feeling of numbness in the affected part.

1st degree: Yellowish-white color, but some softness or resiliency of tissue.
2nd degree: Blisters will rise within 24 hours after thawing of the tissues.
3rd degree: A thin coating of ice appears on the tissue during thawing; within 24 hours of thawing there will be maximum swelling, then discoloration of tissues, and finally decomposition and death of the tissues, with the possibility of gangrene.

The first treatment of frostbite is to *seek shelter*. Do not rub the frostbitten tissues, but apply warmth. Putting the frostbitten parts in warm water should be done as soon as possible, but the temperature of the water should not exceed 107 degrees Fahrenheit. Blisters should not be broken or drained as infection may result and even more drainage may follow. *Never rub a frostbitten area with snow* as more heat will be lost from the body and the skin may be broken or damaged by the rubbing. To prevent frostbite, dress for the weather, be prepared for sudden changes of wind or temperature, avoid sweating, keep clothing dry, avoid touching metal surfaces with the bare skin, avoid head winds, and keep an eye open for the yellow-white appearance of first degree frostbite.

Conserving body heat is the clue to survival in the Arctic. There are three ways when there are no external sources of warmth, such as from a fire:

(1) By proper wear and care of clothing.

(2) By becoming accustomed to keeping the body dry.

(3) By reducing body activity to a minimum, both to conserve heat and to avoid sweating.

Cold weather clothing should have good insulator qualities. Cold weather clothing should be non-compressible and should be resilient. It must be able to resume its original shape after compression in much the way of a sponge rubber ball after pressure has been released.

Clothing must be kept dry. Moisture, oil, dirt and grease cause a loss of insulating qualities of clothing. *The first rule of survival is to keep dry.* Water conducts heat away from the body about 20 times as fast as dry, still air. Snow and frost should be brushed off cothing frequently to keep the clothing as dry as possible, especially when standing near a fire or when entering a shelter or house (where warmth will melt the snow or ice). Wet underclothing (from sweating) is deadly in polar regions. If you get too warm during exertion and start to sweat, then clothing should be loosened for ventilation, some of the clothing should be taken off, or the level of activity should be reduced. Socks should be kept dry and should be changed frequently as perspiration of the feet destroys the insulating quality of the socks.

Clothing must not be compressed. Compression reduces the thickness of materials and reduces the volume of insulating air. Where compression of clothing is greatest, such as on the bottom of the feet (between the shoe sole and the feet), and in the sleeping bag where contact is made with the shoulders, buttocks and feet, there should be greater thickness and protection of insulating materials. Tight gloves and tight footgear are especially dangerous and should be avoided.

The best-fitting garments are those that allow about one-fourth of an inch of dead space between each layer.

Arctic cold and windchill are the greatest hazards. A wind of only 10 miles per hour can freeze human tissue that is exposed in 60 seconds if the temperature is as low as minus 40 degrees Fahrenheit. Outer garments must be windproof in order to eliminate this wind chilling.

Needles and string should be parts of every emergency kit in the arctic for the repair of clothing and the drying of clothing (string or its equivalent as a clothesline).

frostbite

Pruitt, Francis W. "Management of Frostbite in the Korean War," Nebraska State Medical Journal, 39: 3–8, (No. 1), January 1954.

Colonel Francis W. Pruitt, director of the Department of Medicine of the Walter Reed Army Hospital, reports that there were 46,000 cold-injury casualties among the American forces in Europe during the winter of 1944-45. Based on an average of fifty hospital days per patient, it has been estimated that this was a military loss equivalent to the removal of 12 infantry divisions from combat for fifty days.

An estimated 5,000 cold-injury cases occurred in Korea the first winter. There were 1,010 such injuries during the winter of 1951-52, and only 281 in the winter of 1952-53.

At the Osaka Army Hospital in Japan, frostbite casualties were classified in four major categories: (1) redness, tingling, and burning, approximately 17 percent; (2) redness with blisters or vesicles, 34 percent; (3) death of tissue through the skin and into the subcutaneous tissue, 44 percent; and (4) death of all tissue, including bone gangrene and loss of tissue, approximately 6 percent.

Studies have indicated that, once a part of the body has been frozen, best results can be brought about by:

(1) Rapid thawing at a temperature of 86 to 89 degrees F.

(2) The early use of heparin

(3) Avoidance of tobacco

(4) The beginning of medical treatment and hospital care involving bed rest, relief from pain, penicillin, and dictary support, as well as other measures

(5) Allowing a maximum time for tissue regeneration before the decision to amputate is reached

frostbite as a military problem

Lewis, R.B. *"Local Cold Injury—Frostbite," Military Surgeon, 110: 25—41, (No. 1), January 1952.*

Lieutenant Colonel R. B. Lewis of the Medical Corps of the United States Air Force reports that *frostbite, the most severe form of local cold injury, is, in the main, a military problem.*

During World War II frostbite was a major cause of illness in combat ground troops. During the . . . Korean conflict thousands of ground-force personnel suffered frostbite injuries, and many of these were permanently lost as combatants.

The manner in which cold causes injury is not well understood. Two possibilities readily suggest themselves: first, that the tissue injury is caused by damage to the blood vessels, and, second, that the injury is due to the direct action of cold on tissue cells.

The best evidence indicates that frostbite causes injury by acting directly upon the cells. It appears that changes in the blood vessels following frostbite are of secondary importance.

The only curative method which has been universally successful has been that of rapid rewarming of frostbitten tissue. Treatment which has been directed at the blood vessels has given inconsistent results in the hands of various investigators.

Evidence indicates that the damage from frostbite is done at the time of cold injury and that the ultimate injury is a result of three factors: (1) the exposure temperature, (2) the length of time of exposure, and (3) the medium (generally water, air, or metal) conducting heat away from the part of the body involved.

protection of feet immersed in cold water

Spealman, Clair R. "Protection of Feet Immersed in Cold Water," United States Naval Medical Bulletin, 46: 169-78, (No. 2), February 1946.

Clair R. Spealman, United States Naval Reserve, reports on experiments conducted with human subjects who immersed their feet in cold water.

Prolonged immersion of feet in cold water results in damage to blood vessels, nerves and muscles. This condition is commonly called immersion foot and appears to be very similar to trench foot. Injury is due to cold primarily, but interference with return of the blood from the feet by dependency, immobility, or tight clothing is probably a contributory factor.

As a consequence of this study it was shown that swelling, pain, and increased blood flow to the feet occur quickly when the extremities are maintained in cold water at temperatures below 12 to 14 degrees Centigrade. Serious injury does not occur rapidly at these temperatures, however. Feet maintained at an average temperature of 12 degrees Centigrade for 30 hours recovered quickly.

It was shown that very large quantities of insulating materials were needed to prevent immersion foot if exposure is sufficiently prolonged. *Keeping the body warm aided greatly in keeping the feet warm.* Foot exercises also elevated foot temperatures and helped in lymphatic and venous flow. Petrolatum did not appear to give any great protection to feet immersed in cold water.

16
bites and stings

More people die from the stings of bees, wasps, hornets and yellow jackets than from snakebites in the United States. The possibility of anaphylactic shock in sensitive persons stung by winged insects represents a critical challenge for the first aider, but "bee sting" kits, if available, may permit him to meet such a challenge. The bites of dogs carry the potential of rabies, the bites of snakes the hazard of tissue destruction, infection, dissolution of certain blood cells, and the poisoning of nerve tissue, and the bites of certain spiders carry hazards that can be countered only by medical treatment.

The first aider has the responsibility for distinguishing fact from fiction so that he may act intelligently and swiftly for the victims of bites and stings.

anaphylactic reactions to stings

Silverglade, Alex. *"Epinephrine Aerosol for Insect Sting Reactions," Journal of the American Medical Association, 214: 763, (No. 4), October 26, 1970.*

A physician of Northridge, California, in defending the use of the *inhalation of epinephrine spray* into the lungs *in the treatment of severe reactions to insect stings,* points out that only enough of this chemical needs to be absorbed to give relief to symptoms and *to prevent anaphylactic shock,* and that the injection of epinephrine will merely add more than is needed.

Previous medical experience has shown that epinephrine aerosols delivered from pressurized cartridges are effective in the treatment of anaphylactic reactions.

Dr. Silverglade believes that *the ease and speed with which an epinephrine aerosol (spray) can be given,* plus the rapid absorption from the lungs even in the presence of circulatory collapse, justifies its use for serious reactions to allergens and insect bites.

[The *availability of first aid kits with spray preparations* for insect stings that produce anaphylactic shock reactions may well save a human life, whereas the first aider would be unqualified and reluctant in most cases to give an intravenous or subcutaneous injection, even if the necessary equipment were available.— Ed.]

deaths from stings and bites

Parrish, Henry M. *"Analysis of 460 Fatalities from Venomous Animals in the United States," American Journal of the Medical Sciences, 245: 129-141, (No. 2), February 1963.*

An Associate Professor of the University of Missouri School of Medicine reports that venomous animals and insects are found in every state in the United States. *Over a period of 10 years 460 deaths were recorded in this country.* These deaths occurred in the following order of magnitude:

Rank	Animal or Insect	Deaths
1	Bees	124
2	Rattlesnakes	94
3	Wasps	69
4	Spiders	65
5	Unidentified snakes	31
6	Yellow jackets	22
7	Unknown type of animal or insect	18
8	Hornets	10
9	Scorpions	8
10	Cottonmouth moccasins	8
11	Ants	4
12	Coral snakes	2
13	Cobras*	2

14	Boomslang (snake)*	1
15	Stingray	1
16	Unspecified coelenterata	1
	Total	460

*Not indigenous to the United States

Deaths from stinging insects such as bees, wasps, and hornets *occur with alarming suddenness. Most victims died within 15 to 30 minutes.* The patients die from swelling of the larynx, shock, heart failure, and "stroke." To prevent such sudden deaths the following program is advocated:

(1) Identify and *desensitize* persons who are allergic to the venom of the stinging insects.

(2) Instruct hypersensitive patients to *carry insect allergy first aid kits.*

(3) Encourage such patients to wear light colored clothing and to use protective measures.

(4) Educate the public on this medical problem.

It is estimated that 30,000 to 40,000 persons die from snakebite throughout the world each year. Sixty-four per cent of the persons who died from snakebite in this study did so in 6 to 48 hours after the bite. Only 4 per cent died in less than one hour. *It usually takes several hours for the full toxic effects of a snakebite to be felt;* thus, first aid and anti-venom treatment within the first two hours may be lifesaving. Prompt and vigorous medical care should be sought. Two coral snakebite victims died of respiratory paralysis four and five hours respectively after being bitten. The coral snake neurotoxin usually does not paralyze for an hour or more.

Deaths from venomous animals and insects occurred in 45 of the 48 states in this study. The seven leading states were as follows:

Texas	67 deaths
Georgia	36 deaths
California	32 deaths
Florida	26 deaths

Alabama	25 deaths
North Carolina	21 deaths
Kentucky	20 deaths

Agent	Approximate Time Lapse Until Death
1. Bees, wasps, hornets	15-30 minutes
2. Snakebites	6-48 hours
3. Scorpion stings	12 hours or less
4. Spider bites	12-48 hours
5. Stingray stings (only 1 case)	3 days

brown spider bites

Hershey, Falls B. and Carl E. Aulenbacher. "Surgical Treatment of Brown Spider Bites," Annals of Surgery, 170: 300-308, (No. 2), August 1969.

Two surgeons of St. Louis, Missouri report that *the bite of the brown spider, Loxosceles reculusa, may cause localized gangrene, toxicity and even death.*

Hundreds of brown spider bites are treated in physicians' offices and do not need surgical care, but *if gangrene occurs healing may take many weeks and even months* to occur. In such cases surgery may be advisable.

In this study of 17 patients who went to the hospital with brown spider bites, *12 required surgical operations. Gangrene of the skin* from spider bites was first recognized by the medical profession in Chile in 1937. It was not until 1958 that medical investigators in the United States recognized that brown spider bites could cause the death of surrounding tissue, and not until 1961 was it discovered that this spider could cause anemia from the destruction of red blood cells. Since then deaths have been reported in the medical literature from brown spider bites.

Now, *it is known* from animal studies that would not have been possible with humans that *the venom injected by the brown spider may cause the death of tissue and the destruction of red blood cells. It contains a chemical that permits its rapid spread through living tissues.*

After a brown spider bite, nausea, vomiting, chills, aches and pains, and a feeling of illness may develop within 12 to 24 hours in humans. Destruction of red blood cells, blood in the urine, anemia and kidney failure may develop in 12 to 24 hours after severe bites. The most severe and fatal reactions occur in children. A rash may appear on the body after 12 to 24 hours and may last for days.

Loxosceles reculusa, the dark brown spider, has *a violin-shaped mark* on the head and chest. The spider, so far, has been found in Southern California, Texas, and other southwestern states.

In humans, secondary infections are apt to appear in the gangrenous tissue in a few days. At first, only a stinging or itching sensation may be apparent, but after a few hours a painful, red area appears and a red rash may develop. *Severe pain, hemorrhage and discoloration after 48 hours suggests impending death of surrounding tissue.* Infection will occur as long as dead tissue remains. The best treatment is the giving of corticosteroids (to reduce inflammation), antibiotic drugs (to reduce infection) and surgery (to remove dead tissue). Healing cannot occur until the dead tissue is removed. *Surgery is not advised until two to five days after dead tissue appears,* and sometimes later.

black widow spider poisoning

Taussig, Barrett L., and Aaron Hendin. "Black Widow Spider Poisoning," Missouri Medicine, 52: 714-16 (No. 9), September 1955.

Barrett L. Taussig, M.D., and Aaron Hendin, M.D., of St. Louis, Missouri report that the black widow spider (Latrodectus mactans) is widely distributed in the Ohio and Mississippi valleys as well as in the southern states and the Pacific coastal region. [This spider is found in all states.— Ed.] A summary of black widow spider bites made in 1945 showed that from the years 1726 to 1943 a total of 1,291 such cases had been reported in the medical literature, with 55 deaths.

Black widow spiders are occasionally seen in lumber piles, trash heaps, dark corners of woodsheds and garages, and, perhaps most frequently, in outdoor privies.

The poison of the black widow spider, which produces bodily symptoms, is a toxalbumen which is discharged through a duct opening near the tip of the clawlike structure with which the spider seizes its prey.

The signs and symptoms following the bite of the black widow are characteristic, though difficulty in diagnosis may be encountered if the history of the bite cannot be obtained. The severity of the symptoms is related to the amount of venom injected and to the size of the victim. From 15 minutes to two hours following the initial pain of the bite there is onset of severe muscular pain, often starting in the groin and spreading centrifugally to involve the entire body. The pain is excruciating and is often most severe in the abdomen and back. The most striking physical findings include the apparent marked agony of the patient, his inability to sit still or lie down, and the extreme boardlike rigidity of the abdomen, which, however, is not tender to palpation. Other symptoms and findings which have been described but are not invariable include convulsions, sensation of pressure in the chest, vomiting, excessive perspiration and salivation, delirium, and insomnia. The acute symptoms usually subside in from six to forty-eight hours, but in severe cases may last for several days.

The opiates and analgesics have been noteworthy in their relative ineffectiveness in relieving symptoms. The use of intravenous calcium salts has become fairly standard as a therapeutic method, and immediate relief of pain following its use has been described. It is generally agreed that the best and only specific treatment is the use of antivenin (Antivenin *Lactrodectus mactans,* Sharp and Dohme) in dosage of 2.5 cc., deep intramuscularly. A number of patients may require an additional dose. In this article Drs. Taussig and Hendin report a case of black widow spider poisoning in which the patient failed to respond to all nonspecific measures, but made a rapid and complete recovery following the use of specific antiserum.

the black widow spider

California Department of Public Health. "A Few Notes on the 'Black Widow' Spider and Its Bite," California's Health, 5: 338, (No. 18), March 31, 1948.

California has more cases of black widow spider bites credited to it than any other area of the country.

The so-called black widow spider (Latrodectus mactons) is one of the few varieties in the United States whose bite is known to be poisonous to humans. In 1937, 800 cases with 40 deaths were reported throughout the United States.

"Black widow" is the name given to the spider because of its color and the fallacy that the female always attacks and devours the male after mating. Actually, according to recent observations, the female will attack its male partner only when all other sources of food are gone. The spider does not aggressively attack human beings unless its web is disturbed. It is the action of touching the web which ordinarily causes the spider to attack.

The female of this species is much larger than the male and so much more aggressive that most descriptive matter has been based upon the appearance of the female rather than the male. The black widow spider can be easily recognized by the large round abdomen attached by a slender stalk to the front part of the body. The legs and body are a glossy black and on the front surface of the abdomen there is a rich red marking consisting of a rectangular bar from the center of which extends an inverted triangle. The red marking is shaped somewhat like an hour glass and stands out in striking contrast to the surrounding black.

When an individual is bitten by the spider, dramatically sudden and alarmingly severe toxic symptoms result. The first sensation following a bite resembles that of a prick of a very sharp needle. The area becomes blanched followed by reddening with a throbbing lancinating pain. The pain spreads centrally toward the body. If the bite is on the finger the pain spreads up the arm to the chest during the first hour following the bite. Soon there is a profound shock and pain in the abdomen sufficiently severe that cases can easily be mistaken for acute abdominal injury if a history of a spider bite has not been obtained.

An antitoxic serum has been prepared and is said to be effective in treatment. In connection with treatment of these bites, it should be noted that *nothing is gained by applying a tourniquet or by attempting to remove venom from the site of the bite by incision and suction as in bites by poisonous snakes.*

snakebite

Arnold, Robert E. *"Snake Bite!" Journal of the Kentucky Medical Association,* 68: 499-504 ff., (No. 8), August 1970.

A physician of Louisville, Kentucky says that most victims of snakebite are children who are careless or who ignore dangerous areas. (However, four of the five deaths in Kentucky during the last 10 years involved the use of snakes in religious exercises.)

Emergency care given the victim at the site of the accident should have two purposes in mind: 1) to *limit the spread of the venom,* and 2) to *get the patient to the hospital or to a doctor as soon as possible.* Doctor Arnold reports that although there are many procedures such as suction, incision, the use of a tourniquet, cooling, and so on, they contain inherent dangers and should not be used except in a hospital. Valuable time should never be spent in searching for the snake as the antivenin used is the same for all pit vipers (rattlesnakes, moccasins and copperheads) that are responsible for an overwhelming number of snakebites in the United States.

Limitation of the spread of venom can be achieved simply and effectively by applying a splint to the affected arm or leg, and then keeping general body activity to a minimum. Experiments with radioactive-tagged venom show that if the limb is splinted only 22 per cent of the venom will spread within one hour. In this length of time most victims can be taken to a hospital. The victim should be carried if possible.

Incision and suction of the bite wound, if started early and done properly can remove about 50 per cent of the venom, but suction after 30 minutes of elapsed time from being bitten is useless. *Valuable time should not be lost making incisions and starting suction as a first aid measure,* according to Dr. Arnold. A bad situation may become worse. The incision may damage a nerve, may be painful and may make the victim more nervous and hyperactive which would tend to promote the spread of venom. Incision and suction in a hospital by a physician is a safe procedure. The fundamental treatment lies in the prompt use of antivenin.

The venom of the poisonous snake in the United States usually has four effects upon the victim: 1) damages nerve tissue; 2) damages tissue in a way that permits spreading of the venom; 3) digests tissues and 4) produces bleeding. The venom of the reptile is a feeding mechanism rather than a defensive one, says Dr. Arnold. Venom is most effective against rodents, rabbits, frogs and comparable animals which die almost immediately. The prey is swallowed whole and is digested from the inside of the animal by the injected venom. Snakes differ in the amount of the four factors in their venom. The Eastern Diamondback (Crotalus Adamantheus) has the highest concentration of digestive factors and the Mojave Rattlesnake (Crotalus Scutulatus Scutalatus) has the highest concentration of the neurotoxic factor.

Coral snake venom is almost entirely paralytic (neurotoxic) in action. There is no tissue reaction and the pain is only that of the fangs. Symptoms are usually delayed for several hours and the physician may be lulled into a false sense of security in his treatment. Later, apprehension, giddiness, the drooping of eyelids (from muscle paralysis), lethargy, nausea, vomiting and weakness can be expected. Convulsions may occur and paralysis, including respiratory paralysis, may also come. However, some completely paralyzed patients have recovered, so the effects appear to be reversible. Coral antivenin treatment is the key to recovery. The antivenin is not effective against the Arizona Coral Snake, but Dr. Arnold says no deaths have ever occurred from the bite of this snake.

Dr. Arnold says the most common errors in the treatment of

snakebite are not having enough antivenin and giving it by intramuscular injection instead of intravenous. In other words, adequate amounts of antivenin should be used by the physician and should be injected into a blood vessel. Radioactive studies of tagged antivenin have shown that if the injection is made by vein that within two hours 85 per cent of the antivenin will be at the site of the bite, whereas if the injection is made into a muscle only about six per cent of the antivenin will reach the bite area within two hours. The doctor needs to keep a syringe of adrenalin loaded in case of an anaphylactic (allergic shock) reaction to the antivenin.

Histamines, cortisone, alcohol should not be used. They have no beneficial effects. Antihistamines act in a way that enhances the effect of the venom; cortisone interferes with the antigen-antibody reaction between the venom and the antivenin, and alcohol is a depressant and may enhance the speed of spread of venom.

Dr. Arnold strongly urges that *the tourniquet and ice treatment of snakebite should not be used unless the decision has been made to sacrifice the bitten limb* in order to save a life. He reports that this popular form of treatment advocated in 1950 has resulted in many unnecessary amputations and should be condemned. If used, a permit from the patient for amputation should be secured before treatment is started, according to this physician.

facts and fictions about snakebite

Parrish, Henry M. "Venomous Snakebites: Fiction Versus Fact," Journal of the Mississippi State Medical Association, 10: 462-465, (No. 10), October 1969.

A national authority on snakebite, of the School of Medicine, University of South Dakota, observes that *there is a vast amount of misinformation about snakebite accidents.* He discusses these inaccurate beliefs in the following terms.

Fiction: Snakes kill more people annually in the United States than any other venomous animals.

Fact: Snakes are not the most dangerous venomous animals. Of 460 deaths, *bees, wasps, yellow jackets and hornets killed 229 people.* Snakes killed 138, spiders 65, scorpions 8, venomous marine animals 2, and with 18 deaths the venomous animal was unidentified.

Fiction: Most snakes in the United States are venomous and dangerous.

Fact: Only about 10 per cent of the species of snakes native to the United States are venomous.

Fiction: The most dangerous venomous snake in the United States is the coral snake.

Fact: The coral snake, drop for drop, has the most lethal venom, but he produces a small amount of venom, has short fangs, is not very aggressive, is native in only 11 states and bites only 20 to 25 persons per year. In a study of 138 snakebite deaths in the U.S. only 2 were caused by coral snakes. *Large rattlesnakes are the most venomous snakes in this country.*

Fiction: A cottonmouth can't bite a person while under water.

Fact: He can. He often feeds on fish, turtles, frogs and salamanders which he may bite and capture underwater. Numberous case histories of bites of humans by cottonmouths under water are in the medical records.

Fiction: Texas has the highest annual snakebite rate in the United States.

Fact: About 1,400 snakebites do occur in Texas each year, but Texas has a large population. In terms of bites per 100,000 population the rates (rounded to the nearest whole number) are as follows: North Carolina, 19; Arkansas 17; Texas 15; Georgia 13; West Virginia 11; Mississippi 11 and Louisiana 10. *Death rates for snakebite are highest in Arizona, Georgia, Florida, Alabama and South Carolina.* Then comes Texas.

Fiction: Everyone bitten by a venomous snake will be poisoned.

Fact: About 30 per cent of the persons bitten by venomous snakes do not develop signs of vernom poisoning, because of indirect hits by the fangs, because the snake may have emptied his venom sac from recent feedings, because of a broken fang or for some other reason.

Fiction: A high percentage of persons bitten by venomous snakes will die. *Fact:* Although about 6,680 persons are bitten by venomous snakes each year in the United States, only about 14 will die. *Less than one-fourth of 1 per cent of persons bitten by venomous snakes die.* Most of those who died were guilty of delay in seeking medical care or received inadequate amounts of antivenin. *Fiction:* Most snakebites occur in the woods or in uninhabited places. *Fact: About 55 per cent of the copperhead bites occur in the victim's own yard, under or on the porch or in the patio* of a building. *About 60 per cent of the bites of a cottonmouth occur in or near water;* 20 per cent are in the victim's own yards (probably located near water). *About 35 per cent of rattlesnakes bites occur in fields and on farms away from the house, 27 per cent occur in the victim's own yard, 14 per cent occur under buildings* and 5 per cent on or near roads. Only about 13 per cent occur in the woods. Most coral snake bites occur while people are handling snakes, picking up boards or logs from the ground or while the victims are working in the garden.

Fiction: Most snakebites occur at night because snakes feed at night.

Fact: Snakebites occur when *people* are active. *About 86 per cent of snakebite accidents* occur between 6 a.m. and 9 p.m.; thus, most *occur in the daytime.*

Fiction: Snakebites occur below the knee.

Fact: About 60 per cent of the bites of venomous snakes are inflicted on the lower extremities, but *38 per cent occur on the upper extremities* and the remaining 2 per cent on the head, face, neck or trunk.

Fiction: Most persons who died from venomous snakebite will die in the first two hours after the bite.

Fact: It usually takes several hours for the full effects of the venom of a snake to take effect because much of the venom is deposited in the tissues of the victim. *Of 138 deaths from snakebite, only 4 per cent died within one hour and only 17 per cent died within 6 hours. About 64 per cent died 6 to 48 hours after the bite.* Any snakebite victim who can obtain medical care within 2 hours of a bite has a very good chance for survival.

Fiction: One bite by a venomous snake will provide permanent immunity against subsequent bites.

Fact: Frequent injections of venom are necessary to maintain immunity. If these injections stop, immunity declines to low levels within about 3 months. Antivenin treatment after a bite is a much more rational approach to the saving of life.

Fiction: Venomous bites are more deadly to children than to adults.

Fact: The greatest number of deaths from snakebite are found for adults in the age group 60 to 69 years of age; *other diseases, such as heart disease, are probably contributing factors to the higher death rate.* Children, theoretically in greater hazard because they would receive more venom in proportion to blood volume and body size, do get approximately the same amount of antivenin that adults receive if they obtain medical treatment. *Persons 70 years and older have about four times the death rate of children from venomous bites.*

snakebite

Parrish, Henry M., Stanley L. Silberg and John C. Goldner. "Snakebite: A Pediatric Problem," Clinical Pediatrics, 4: 237-241, (No. 4), April 1965.

Two physicians and a public health worker report that *less than 1 per cent of the persons who are bitten by a poisonous snake in the United States will die.* About 7,000 persons are bitten annually in the United States by venomous reptiles, but in a ten-year period there were only 138 snakebite deaths. Children and young adults comprise about 40 to 60 per cent of all the victims. In the 10-year period from 1950 to 1959 snakebites were reported from every state except Maine in the Continental United States.

Pit vipers are responsible for more than 99 per cent of all poisonous snakebites in the United States. Coral snakes are responsible for the remainder. Rattlesnakes, copperheads, and cottonmouths are pit vipers.

Pit vipers have a characteristic pit between the eye and the nostril on each side. *They also have elliptical pupils and two well-developed fangs* that protrude when the mouth is open. Rattlesnakes also have rattles attached to their tails. A single row of subcaudal plates is diagnostic.

Harmless snakes do not have pits and they lack fangs, although they do have teeth. In addition they have round rather than elliptical pupils. Harmless snakes also have a double row of subcaudal plates. *It is important to make a distinction between a poisonous snakebite and venation (snake venom poisoning).* This is more important than being able to identify poisonous and harmless snakes because 1) often the victim will not see the snake that has bitten him; 2) many times the snake will not be captured or killed; 3) it is possible for a poisonous snake to bite someone without injecting enough venom to produce poisoning (venenation).

Puncture wound and *pain* are the two local signs of venenation along with *swelling* (edema) and *inflammation* (erythema). *Usually at least three of these four signs of venenation are present.* One or more fang wounds are necessary to produce venenation. If swelling and redness have not developed within 4 hours after a snakebite it can be concluded the victim does not have a pit viper venenation. If the bite is poisonous it may take 12 to 24 hours before the swelling stops spreading.

Signs and symptoms that are more general include those of shock; nausea; vomiting; diarrhea; blood in the stool (intestinal discharges); numbness, tingling, and strange feelings in the hands or feet, coma, convulsions and motor or respiratory paralysis. Anemia and disturbances of blood clotting may occur also.

The amount of venenation provides a guide for the amount of antivenin that may be needed for treatment. Bites are classified as follows:

Grade 0: (No venenation). Fang or tooth marks may be present, but there is a minimum of pain and any swelling or redness is less than one inch in circumference. There are no general or systemic involvements or symptoms.

Grade 1: (Minimal venenation). Fang or tooth marks are present with severe pain and from one to five inches of surrounding swelling and inflammation within 12 hours after the bite. There are no general symptoms affecting the whole body.

Grade 2: (Moderate venenation). Fang or tooth marks are present with severe pain. There is swelling and inflammation over an area of about six to twelve inches within twelve hours after the bite. In addition, some general symptoms are present such as nausea, vomiting, giddiness, shock or neurological symptoms.

Grade 3: (Severe venenation). Fang or tooth marks are present with severe pain. *More* than 12 inches of swelling and inflammation occur within 12 hours after the bite and the general symptoms such as nausea, vomiting, shock or neurological effects are accentuated.

First Aid for Snakebite. A tourniquet should be applied to the bitten arm or leg at a point several inches from the bite (On the side closest to the heart). As the swelling spreads the tourniquet should be shifted to keep ahead of the swelling. The purpose is to slow down or impede the spread of venom. Tourniquets lengthen the survival time, but do not necessarily prevent death. The tourniquet should not stop the arterial circulation and it should be released every 10 to 15 minutes for a minute or two. Incision and suction to remove venom is helpful if it is done within the first 120 minutes after the snakebite. The sooner incision and suction is done the more effective it is. Suction cups in snakebite kits are effective in the removal of venom.

Treatment includes the first aid procedures and "the three A's" (antivenin, antibiotics, and antitoxin (or toxoid) for tetanus). For more serious bites the antivenin needs to be given by vein. Injections of antivenin in the arm or buttocks are satisfactory for Grade 1 venenations. The smaller the body (as in a child) the larger the antivenin injection. Germs are present in both the mouths and the venoms of snakes and it is for this reason that antibiotics are used to prevent infections. It is for this reason that antitoxin or toxoid for the prevention of tetanus is recommended also.

animal bites and rabies

Jones, Ronald C. "Rabies: Present Attitudes," Postgraduate Medicine, 43: 141-14 (No. 3), March 1968.

An Assistant Professor of Surgery at the University of Texas Southwestern Medical School at Dallas reports that *about 2,000,000 persons are bitten by animals yearly and that about half a million of these bites are by dogs.*

The dog that bites without apparent cause or provocation should be considered a mad dog (rabid). Mad dogs are apt to move about without purpose or object, snapping and drooling. Their vocal cords are paralyzed. Death of the rabid dog usually occurs within 2 to 5 days. If it is known that a biting dog has been vaccinated against rabies this fact should be ignored, for the rabies vaccine used in dogs is not 100% cent effective.

The immediate first aid care of an animal bite may make the difference between life and death. Free bleeding from the wound should be encouraged. In animals studied by one group of investigators the development of rabies after wound contamination with the rabies vaccine was reduced from about 95 per cent to only 10 per cent when the wound was treated with benzalkonium chloride (Zephiran), Ivory soap, and antirabies serum used singly or in sequence, especially if applied within 3 to 6 hours.

First aid care of an animal bite should consist of thorough irrigation (washing) with large amounts of saline solution (containing salt), cleansing with 20 per cent saline solution, swabbing with a 1 or 2 per cent solution of benzalkonium chloride (Zephiran), debridement (clean-up of the wound by the surgeon or physician) and administration of antibiotics and tetanus toxoid. In wounds that permit adequate application, Zephiran or soap, or both, is considered as effective as, and probably more effective than fuming nitric acid, according to Dr. Jones. *Antiserum applied directly to the wound is remarkably effective in preventing rabies in experimental animals. All soap should be removed before application of Zephiran as it will neutralize the activity of such a compound.* Rabies vaccine should not be given by a physician unless there is a definite indication for its use.

Rabies vaccine prepared in duck embryo has been widely used since it became available in 1957. Neurologic reactions have been reported in only five persons and all recovered with no permanent damage. No deaths have been due to the use of this vaccine. No antibiotic or chemotherapeutic agent has been found to work against rabies, but it may be prevented by the use of antiserum and the rabies vaccine. Of persons bitten by rabid animals not given the antirabies treatment about 50 to 75 per cent will develop rabies. About 40,000 to 60,000 persons receive antirabies vaccine each year.

dog bite

Kruglick, John S. "Dog Bite and Its Complications," Arizona Medicine, 12: 13-15 (No. 1), January 1955.

John S. Kruglick, M.D., of Phoenix, Arizona, says that the treatment of dog bite or the bite of other potentially rabid animals needs clarification in respect to the use of rabies vaccine and the reaction that sometimes occurs from this product.

Dr. Kruglick advocates the following treatment for dog bites or injuries received from other animals of a like nature:

(1) Dog bites (or other animal bites) should be washed for five minutes with soap and should then be treated as the wound demands.

(2) Bites about the neck, face, or hands should be treated immediately. Five injections of rabies vaccine should be given. The dog should be observed, and if he does not develop rabies or run

away, and remains healthy, the use of the vaccine may be discontinued. If the animal develops rabies, then a total of 21 vaccine injections should be given the patient.

(3) Severe bites of the face, neck, and hands should be treated as in the foregoing paragraph, with the addition of immune gamma globulin.

(4) Bites of the trunk and extremities other than the hands should be treated only if the dog is not available for observation or if the observed animal becomes rabid. Fourteen rabies vaccine injections are recommended for a complete course of treatment in these cases.

(5) All patients suffering from dog bites should receive a tetanus booster injection.

(6) Rabies vaccine injections should be stopped if any type of reaction occurs. If it is necessary to continue the injections the patient should be desensitized.

(7) All patients with an allergic history should be carefully watched and those who have received previous treatment with rabies vaccine should be skin-tested for sensitivity.

(8) Although various types of reactions may occur to the rabies vaccine, the patient needs more careful observation in some types than in others. Very close observation of the patient is needed when there is inflammation of the brain as a reaction to the use of the vaccine.

(9) Antihistamines and cortisone have given particularly good results in the treatment of serious types of reactions to the rabies vaccine and should be used as the occasion demands.

(10) Contrary to the beliefs of some people the judicious use of rabies vaccine represents sound medical treatment in dog bite cases. *One must keep in mind that rabies is 100 per cent fatal if it is untreated.*

17
emergencies of vision

The eyes can be damaged in many ways. Some of the more serious dangers to vision may be completely unrelated to an eye injury. Sudden blindness, from whatever cause, must always be considered an emergency that demands immediate attention of a physician and preferably an eye specialist.

For some eye accidents, such as those involving chemical splashing, the first aid procedures used on the spot may be more important than later medical care in the preservation of vision. Prompt, copious, and sustained washing of the chemically-injured eye may save it from blindness.

visual complications from drugs

Leopold, Irving H. "Ocular Complications of Drugs," Journal of the American Medical Association, 205: 631-633, (No. 9), August 26, 1968.

The folly of young people assuming that they know all about the effects of drugs is illustrated in this report by a physician from the Department of Ophthalmology of the Mount Sinai School of Medicine in New York. Dr. Leopold observes that *visual complications from the use of drugs have been observed in medicine for centuries.*

Undesirable and damaging effects on the eyes may be produced by almost all categories of drugs that are given internally by the physician. *All manner of visual disturbances from drugs may occur,* such as blurred vision, disturbed color vision, sensitivity to light, flickerings, flashes and sparks, reduction in visual acuity (the ability to see), eye-muscle weakness or paralysis, degeneration of the retina (the part of the eye that contains the light-receiving cells) and blindness, constriction of the blood vessels of the eye, inflammation of the retina and optic nerve, constriction of the visual field and so on.

[In saving the life of a patient who suffers from a disorder that can be cured or helped with a particular drug, the physician and the patient may both accept the risk that vision may be impaired in some manner or other, but the significance of Dr. Leopold's article for young people considering the use of drugs is profound. If a physician cannot predict the effect of a drug in terms of complications with a particular individual, no young person without medical training can safely assume that he can take *any* drug without the possibility of damage.—Ed.]

All parts of the eye structures may be damaged by drugs, but those parts that appear to be most vulnerable to injury are the conjunctiva, cornea, sclera, lens, retina, optic nerve and the eye muscles.

Drugs given for heart disease, for reduction of body fluids, for infections (such as the antibiotics), the tranquilizing, depressing or stimulating drugs, and many others may all produce injurious effects upon the eyes.

The physician can predict the effects of some drugs on the visual apparatus as the effects may occur within a short time, but other drugs produce damaging effects only after they have been used for a long time. *Many of the effects cannot be predicted* on the basis of clinical experience or animal experiments. All persons who receive drugs internally should be carefully studied in terms of possible effects upon vision, according to this eye specialist.

eye burns and tear gas

Hoffmann, D. H. *"Eye Burns Caused by Tear Gas," British Journal of Ophthalmology, 51: 265-268 (No. 4), April 1967.*

A physician of the Hamburg University School of Medicine in West Germany reports from his experience of treating 50 persons with eye injuries due to tear gas that damage to vision from this source occurs only when the shots from tear gas guns are fired at close range. At long range the tear gas irritant reaches the eyes in gaseous form and *such shots are not dangerous to eyesight.*

It is only when the shot is fired at a distance of about one to six feet from the face of the victim that damage to the eyes may occur. In a tear gas shell the chemical (usually chloracetophenon) is sealed in the cartridge with cork or a layer of wax. When a shot is fired at close range the chemical, the charge, and the sealing substance may all enter the eyeball. Treatment, therefore, must be directed not only at the tear gas chemical but at removal of the solid part infiltrations. Usually, however, most of the damage is of a chemical nature.

Various complications may follow injury from close-range tear gas shots. Destruction of eye tissues, hemorrhage, damage to the optic nerve, secondary glaucoma and cataracts are some of the complications that may occur. Infections and ulcers may occur also.

Loss of vision may vary from almost perfect retention of eyesight to the other extreme of being able to perceive light only. The distance of the shot and the amount of infiltrated substances tend to determine the ultimate amount of loss of vision. When one eye only is affected, the loss of vision tends to be greater, because the distance of the shot is usually very close (so close it affects only one eye).

Little is know about tissue changes due to infiltration of the chemical. It is possible that hydrochloric acid may be set free when chloracetophenon comes in contact with protein, so that death of eye tissues by coagulation may occur.

Some countries forbid tear gas weapons. Penalties have been imposed upon foreign tourists who have taken gas pistols to England. In West Germany the dangerous close-range shots that cause damage to vision were not made by the police, but mainly by antisocial, imprudent, and careless persons. (In West Germany there are no uniform laws on the subject, as each state has its own ruling.)

detachment of the retina

Henry, Morriss M. "Diagnosis of Retinal Detachment," Journal of the Arkansas Medical Society, 63: 104-108 (No. 3), August 1966.

An eye specialist of Fayetteville, Arkansas reports that everyone sees occasional spots in the field of vision for one reason or another.

The sudden onset of spots and flashes of light is one of the first symptoms of a retinal tear or detachment. The patient who reports to his physician or eye doctor that he saw black spots and flashing lights could be nearing total blindness, because *if a retinal tear or hole is not repaired soon after the symptoms occur there may be total loss of vision in the affected eye.*

Any hemorrhage into the vitreous (glassy part of the eyeball) that the physician can observe should alert him to the possibility that his patient may be experiencing the beginning of a torn or detached retina. *Hemorrhage into the eyeball that causes black spots means that some disorder is present. Even a very small hemorrhage should be considered as indicative of a torn retina unless a complete eye examination proves otherwise.*

Flashing lights are probably due to excessive stimulation of the retina (the inner layer or coat of the eye that contains the nerve cells that are sensitive to light) because of a shrinking vitreous. Although a shrinking vitreous is a part of the normal aging process, it may become attached to the retina, possibly as the result of an injury. As the vitreous shrinks it may pull a hole in the retina.

Many patients will date the onset of their retinal detachment to a blow on the head or eye. Most retinal detachments are not ordinarily due to a blow, but a beginning detachment may be made rapidly worse by it and the patient suddenly becomes aware of the loss of vision in his eye. If a person has had a blow to the head or eye and spots and flashes appear, he should report to an eye specialist at once.

All torn parts of the retina must be carefully located and repaired. If one hole is missed, a second operation or treatment will be necessary. Some patients will have more than one hole in the retina. Correction and preservation of vision demands the closing of all torn places.

Reattachment of the retina to the underlying choroid (middle coat of the eyeball that contains blood vessels that supply nutrients and oxygen to the retina) can be expected in about 80 to 90 per cent of the cases of retinal detachment if medical care is sought soon enough. If the retina is not reattached or anchored to the choroid it will continue to peel away with extensive loss of vision or total blindness.

foreign bodies in the eye

Clark, William B. "The Management of Corneal Lesions Following Trauma," Industrial Medicine and Surgery, 32: 47-52, (No. 2), February 1963.

A Professor of Clinical Ophthalmology of the Tulane University School of Medicine says that *the successful treatment of eye injuries depends upon proper first aid care.* The observation of a few fundamental rules in caring for injuries to the cornea of the eye may mean the difference between preservation and loss of vision.

It is well that first aid be *limited* to:

1) Gently removing superficial foreign bodies with a tightly wound cotton applicator moistened with 1:3000 Zephiran;

2) Irrigating the eye with plain water;

3) Covering the eye with a sterile pad;

4) Instructing the patient to keep as quiet as possible, and

5) Referring him to an ophthalmologist.

Accidents to the cornea of the eye do not always cause total loss of vision, but there is so much pain and photophobia that usually the injured person cannot carry on any activity until the eye has recovered from the injury.

Injury to the cornea may result from foreign bodies, burns from heat or chemicals, and exposure to certain irritants.

The degree of injury from a foreign body depends upon: 1) depth of penetration; 2) composition of the penetrating material; 3) temperature of the penetrating material; 4) time until removal and 5) the damage done in any attempts at removal.

In many cases more damage is done in attempted removal than by the foreign body itself. Deep foreign bodies should be removed only by the ophthalmologist.

Most metallic substances do not interact with the cornea, but the exceptions include steel, magnesium, mercury, copper, beryllium and nickel.

A first move by the doctor is to protect against infection by the instillation of antibiotics. Steroids should not be used in any form on a fresh wound. They reduce the victim's resistance to fungus infection, and predispose to infection with the herpes virus that causes the serious dendritic ulcer. Tetanus antitoxin and a booster dose of tetanus toxoid is advisable in penetrating injuries.

Most corneal abrasions heal promptly and a new layer of epithelium may be present after 24 hours, but even the simplest abrasion may cause severe pain and secondary inflammation of the iris.

Injury to the cornea may be caused by contact lenses if they are worn continuously for 12 hours or more, if they are poorly fitted, and if they are chipped or warped. Ulceration and scarring and a deeper keratitis may occur. If contact lenses are discontinued, the cornea usually becomes clear and vision returns to its former level.

Iron or steel may stain the cornea. If the rust deposit causes irritation, reddening and photophobia, it should be removed by the ophthalmologist. Copper deposits may be dissolved after several months, but removal may be necessary.

Inflammation of the cornea may result even two or three months after a bee sting on the outside of the lid. It may take this time for the stinger to migrate through the lid to the under surface. When the inner surface of the lid is exposed the stinger often moves back and disappears and may be very difficult to find.

Caterpillar hairs may cause irritation of the cornea within a few hours. They may migrate slowly through tissue into the anterior chamber and the inflammation may last for two or three months.

Chestnut burs are a fairly common cause of eye injury. The thorns may break off under the surface of the cornea and penetrate more deeply, but may not cause inflammation. Wood is generally well tolerated by the eye.

Of all burns to the cornea those due to alkali are the most serious. Alkali injuries cause nearly seven times as much blindness as retinal detachment. Alkali burns are progressive and serious late complications may develop. *The most important first aid measure is thorough cleansing with water.* If undissolved particles of the alkali are present they should be removed by gentle swabbing.

eye injuries

Christensen, Leonard. "Emergency Management of Ocular Injuries," GP, XXIII: 113-20, (No. 1), January 1961.

A physician of the Department of Ophthalmology of the University of Oregon Medical School in Portland says that the eye presents many peculiarities of anatomy and function that set it aside from all other organs. *Most serious eye injuries should be treated by a specialist.*

Essentially, the eye is a sphere composed of a tough outer nonelastic membrane, the cornea and sclera, which acts as a protection for an inner photosensitive membrane, the retina. In addition to protection, the cornea is also transparent and thus acts as a window and is the major refracting surface for light entering the eye. The retina communicates with the brain via the optic nerve. The optic nerve is not a true nerve, but is an extension of the brain and is incapable of regeneration once it is severed.

The cornea is subject to many injuries because of its exposed position and is often damaged indirectly through injury to adjacent tissues, such as the lids. Corneal injury is particularly serious, since not only its integrity but also its transparency must be maintained.

Some of the more common types of injuries to the eye include:

1) *Lid injuries.* Any lacerations or tears of the lid must be very carefully repaired. The lid is a membrane that must move; when interference with movement occurs, an incapacity is created. Also, because of its prominent position, any deviation in appearance from the opposite lid is usually obvious, constituting a severe cosmetic defect.

2) *Contusion (bruise) of the globe.* Pressure from a blow to the eye is immediately transmitted to all parts of the eye and momentarily may be extremely high. If the pressure is sufficiently great, the globe will explode, rupturing the outer coat. Rupture of the globe is always accompanied by severe loss of vision and a markedly soft eye. Other effects of contusion include detachment of the retina, dislocations of the lens, intraocular hemorrhages, and edema of the retina. For severe ocular contusion, bed rest with binocular dressings for four to five days may help prevent complications.

3) *Superficial lacerations.* Lacerations of the globe most often involve the cornea or the immediately-adjacent tissues. Superficial lacerations are painful and potentially dangerous. They usually occur from a scratch by a fingernail, particularly a baby's nail, or contact with vegetable material such as branches of trees. Immediately after injury, pain, abnormal sensitivity to light, and excessive lacrimation (tearing) are experienced. The symptoms may persist and be made worse by frequent blinking. Treatment consists partly of pressure dressing to inhibit the action of the lids for 12 to 24 hours, and antibiotics may be given.

4) *Deep lacerations.* Deep lacerations present a more complex problem because of potential impairment of vision. Early treatment should be directed largely toward prevention of infection. Induced paralysis of the lids may be desirable until the wound can be treated by a specialist.

5) *Corneal foreign body.* This is one of the most common types of eye injury. The victim experiences sudden pain, followed by a persistent foreign body sensation, tearing, and sensitivity to light. Treatment usually consists of removal under local anesthetic. Some metallic foreign bodies induce a rust ring around the edge of the wound.

This ring is difficult to remove initially, but usually separates itself from the cornea in 24 hours and may then be easily removed.

6) *Intraocular foreign body.* This is a serious accident, often involving a small piece of steel which breaks loose at a high velocity from the force of a blow with a chisel or hammer. These fragments may pass entirely through the eye. The victim experiences immediate pain and discomfort which often subside rapidly. Often examination does not reveal a point of entry or other evidence of penetration. Subsequent inflammation is almost invariable. A diagnosis may be established quickly by x-rays; this procedure should be performed whenever the possibility of an intraocular foreign body is considered. Extraction must be performed very carefully.

7) *Ultraviolet burns.* These burns may occur from exposure to sun, ultraviolet lamps and arc welding. Most ultraviolet burns of the cornea are superficial and ordinarily are fully healed within 12 hours. A firm pressure dressing to fix the lids and prevent rubbing on the cornea from blinking may be advisable in some cases.

8) *Chemical burns.* Chemical burns are becoming an increasing problem because of greater exposure of the population to various caustic chemicals. Acid burns tend to be less destructive than base burns. Bases penetrate deeply within the tissues and ultimately create far greater tissue destruction. *The immediate treatment of chemical burns* consists of copious and prolonged irrigation with water. No time should be lost searching for a neutralizing agent.

alkali burns of the eye

Dennis, Richard H. "A Simple Procedure for Treatment of Alkali Burns of the Eye," Journal of the Maine Medical Association, 45: 32ff., (No. 2), February 1954.

Richard H. Dennis, M.D., of Waterville, Maine, reminds us that alkali burns of the eye can cause disastrous permanent disability much greater than burns that are caused by most other chemicals.

This is apparently because the alkali combines chemically with tissue mucoproteins in such a way as to prolong the burning action.

The aims of treatment of alkali burns should be the elimination of the toxic substance, its dilution and neutralization with whatever suitable substance we may have at our command, and prevention of secondary infection.

The first part of the course of treatment begins at the site of the accident. *The eye should be copiously irrigated with whatever bland irrigating substance can be found immediately available. This is usually water.*

Every alkali burn should be considered a hospital case, if possible, even if this is only for the remainder of the day on which the accident has occurred. Here the eye should also be irrigated with copious amounts of fluid. This is usually normal saline because this is immediately available in the hospital. Anesthesia is then used in the eye and all particles of devitalized tissue as well as of alkaline substance are removed. Irrigation is carried out with normal saline every fifteen minutes for the entire first day and is then cut down to half-hour intervals during the night. The next day the irrigations can be reduced to hourly intervals. Further reduction depends upon the rapidity of the improvement of the individual burn, but after the fourth day further irrigation is of little value.

Neutralization can be carried out as soon as the patient is seen by the doctor. *If nothing more than a weak acid such as household vinegar is used, in the proportion of one teaspoon to a quart of water, this will be of value.* This can be carried out during the first day as part of the irrigating solution. Neutral ammonium salts are almost always unavailable.

To prevent secondary infections which may result in subsequent scarring and adhesions, an antibiotic is used concurrently with the irrigation. Terramycin drops, aureomycin ophthalmic solution, or even sulfadiazine may be employed at hourly intervals the first day, then every two hours thereafter until the eye is well healed. It must be remembered that the concentration of the antibiotic has to be maintained at a high constant level to be of value.

The use of egg membrane, which can be easily obtained, has been suggested in very severe cases to prevent adhesions. The egg membrane is laid over the eye in such a way as to separate raw, opposing surfaces of the eye structures.

eye emergencies in industry

Knapp, Arthur Alexander. *"Eye Emergencies in Industry,"* Journal of the American Medical Association, 146: 12-16, (No. 1), May 5, 1951.

Arthur Alexander Knapp, M.D., of New York City, says that eye emergencies in industry have assumed a tremendous importance.

About 80 percent of the accidents to the eye in industry are due to flying bodies, whereas about 8 percent are due to tools or parts of machinery, 7 percent to splashing liquids, 2.5 percent to explosions, 2 percent to falls, and less than 1 percent to infections.

In the mechanical industries, more foreign bodies or flying particles enter the left eye than the right eye. This is apparently due to the fact that most people are right-handed and work at such as angle that the left eye is more exposed to danger.

When flying objects enter the eyeball, there is need for highly specialized medical care, which should be rendered as quickly as possible. In the case of chemical burns to the eye, there should be extensive dilution and washing out of the chemical with water. As soon as possible following the injury, the damaged area should be flushed continuously with water for many minutes, or the patient's head should be periodically immersed in a pail of water. Mechanical removal of chemical substances from the eye should supplement the washing, whenever possible. The important point in giving first aid for this type of injury is that flushing with water should be carried on zealously for a long period of time. Medical treatment must follow the rendering of first aid.

Sometimes medical care may be sought for what appears to be an eye emergency but which may actually represent an allergic condition. There may be marked swelling and redness of the eyelids or of the eyeball, with sensitivity to light, itching, and a slight discharge. The absence of bacterial infection, the abrupt appearance of the disorder, and the disappearance of the symptoms on removal of an offending substance, coupled with certain laboratory evidence, may make diagnosis of the allergy relatively simple. Immediate temporary relief by proper medical treatment should confirm the diagnosis.

18
dental injuries

Blows to the mouth, of whatever origin, often cause prompt and extensive bleeding because of the rich blood supply of the tissues involved. Parents of children with mouth injuries may rush their children for medical care, the wounds involved may heal rapidly, especially with good treatment, but the longer and more serious potential of injury to the teeth may be overlooked by the parents unless the physician urges dental attention. In other words, dental injuries can and do occur that may not be apparent in accidents.

In accidents involving the mouth the competent dentist should always be consulted. If teeth are actually knocked loose they should be taken to the dentist along with the patient, for it may be possible for the teeth to be placed in position again for the rendering of years of future service.

persistent bleeding after tooth extraction

Poswillo, D. E. "The Emergency Treatment of Dental Bleeders in Medical Practice," New Zealand Medical Journal, 66: 522-525 (No. 420), August 1967.

The Senior Oral Surgeon of the North Canterbury Hospital Board of Christchurch, New Zealand recommends that whenever a physician is called by a patient who is bleeding after a dental extraction that he should advise the patient to:

(1) Eat a substantial meal of scrambled eggs and coffee if no food has been consumed for six hours.

(2) Wash all blood off the face and hands after eating and rinse out the mouth well with warm salt water. Any hanging clots should be freed with gauze or linen if necessary. The patient should then sit up in bed supported by a pillow and bite firmly on a pad of gauze or cotton wool, 2 x 2 inches when compressed. This pad must be held tightly between the jaws over the bleeding socket with firm biting pressure for a minimum of 20 minutes without

being removed. Saliva may be swallowed normally during this procedure.

(3) If the bleeding has not stopped after the foregoing procedures then the patient should call the physician again within 10 minutes after the pack has been removed if bleeding continued.

The nature of the blood loss after dental extraction is important. Dental bleeding of a minor nature often involves expectoration of copious amounts of thin, blood-stained saliva. This kind of bleeding may continue for as long as 24 hours after extraction, but it seldom needs emergency attention. Troublesome bleeding after the extraction of a tooth may involve the loss of large clots of blood. *When large clots are expectorated there is need for immediate medical attention.*

In more than 60 per cent of dental hemorrhage the bleeding point is in the upper molar socket area. The application of a pressure pad to this area after removal of loose or protruding clots generally produces a stable clot that is level with the margins of the socket. If a pressure pad applied by the patient does not stop the bleeding, the physician may have to clean out the area of imperfect clots and suture the socket to pull the soft tissue margins together. Other measures may be judged to be necessary also by the examining dental surgeon. After arrest of the hemorrhage a suitable sedative may be prescribed to assure the patient of release from tension and to provide restful sleep for the remainder of the night. Sutures and sedation are the main lines of treatment for the patient with a dental hemorrhage. If these measures fail, then the patient should be transferred to a hospital for investigation and treatment.

treatment of injured teeth

Down, C. H. "The Treatment of Permanent Incisor Teeth of Children Following Traumatic Injury," Australian Dental Journal, 2: 9-24 (No. 1, February 1957.

C. H. Down, D.D.Sc., professor of dentistry at the University of Melbourne, Australia, reports that injuries to the permanent incisor teeth of children have become so frequent during recent years that a knowledge of their treatment is essential to every dentist.

A study of 329 patients who were treated at the Dental School of the University of Melbourne and the Dental Hospital of Melbourne because of injuries to their teeth showed that approximately 80 per cent of such injuries occurred to the upper central incisors, and that approximately 60 per cent of the injuries occurred during the years when the roots of the teeth were not fully developed.

In this group of 329 patients a total of 471 teeth were injured.

In this study it was found that injuries to the teeth may result in fracture of the crown, death of the pulp, calcification of the pulp, fracture of the root, partial dislodgement of the tooth from its socket, depression of the tooth into its socket, total dislodgement of the tooth from its socket, or extensive damage requiring extraction of the tooth.

In this study only nine of 464 damaged teeth had to be extracted. Three of these extractions were due to the fracture of the root in close proximity to the gum margin, one to gross displacement with complete dislodgement of two other teeth, four to acute inflammation of the supporting dental structures, and one to an unknown reason.

In this study the small number of teeth that had to be extracted is encouraging and indicates that it is possible to obtain successful results in a very high proportion of injuries to the teeth. *On the other hand, the study suggests that treatment should be carried out as soon as possible after the receipt of the injury and preferably within 24 hours of its occurrence.*

Following injury to a tooth the mouth should be irrigated with warm salt solution or some comparable preparation, and if lacerations or cuts are present they should be treated with some suitable antiseptic. An appropriate sedative dose of aspirin may also be indicated.

Every injured tooth and the nearby teeth should be examined by x-ray to determine evidence of fracture of the root and the degree of development of the root, as well as possible retention of a portion of the root if the tooth has been totally dislodged from its socket. Evidence of the degree of development of the root is important because it has a bearing on subsequent treatment.

The dentist must also examine the teeth carefully to see if there is an exposure of the pulp. In some cases exposure is evident and in others a pinkish tinge suggests a near exposure. Vitality tests of the pulps of nearby, apparently uninjured and opposing teeth must be made, because death of the pulp is more frequent in teeth without fracture of the crown than in teeth with fractured crowns and in teeth with incompletely developed roots, according to Dr. Down. The mobility of the injured teeth and the approximating teeth must also be tested and recorded. The alignment of the teeth in the arch must be checked to notice any displacement, but the patient or the patient's parents should be questioned about the position of the teeth before the accident.

Steps should be taken at once to protect the vital pulp from injury by heat or cold and against additional infection.

Following careful examination and diagnosis of the severity of the injury, the dentist must then, of course, embark upon a program of treatment.

dental injuries

Morvay, Leonard S. "The Physician and Dental and Jaw Injuries," Industrial Medicine and Surgery, 24: 307-08, (No. 7), July 1955.

A dentist from Newark, New Jersey has reported to the Academy of Medicine that the average physician can rarely make a reasonably accurate determination of the percentage of jaw disability following the completed treatment for a jaw fracture.

Understandably, *the dentist, with his special training, is better equipped to render first aid in the case of a jaw injury* than is the physician, but if a dentist is not immediately available, there are certain emergency procedures that the physician should undertake.

Basic emergency treatment for jaw fractures is application of a four-tail bandage. Treatment is similar to that employed for fractures of the extremities; it includes periodic ice packing, sedation, and the administration of antibiotics.

Only the dentist should be permitted to provide definitive treatment for jaw fractures and complicated, extensive loss of teeth; also, he should be brought into the picture as soon as it is possible.

When trauma to the teeth and surrounding tissues occurs, every effort should be made to preserve the involved teeth even though they may be so extremely mobile that removal appears to be the only treatment indicated. The immobilization of loose teeth by interdental wiring, followed, if necessary, by the application of a splint, stabilizes teeth within a week or 10 days after the accident even though the teeth may have been extremely loose immediately following the trauma.

Even completely dislodged teeth, when recovered, immediately sterilized and replaced in their sockets, become solidly attached to the alveolus in many cases. With modern treatment these teeth, once thought to be permanently lost, will serve their owners long and well if they are replaced in the socket void within 12 hours. The sooner they are replaced, the more favorable the prognosis.

The victim of a jaw injury must not be permitted to test the looseness of involved teeth by digital pressure, since this retards the natural reparative process which begins immediately after injury. No food which would put a strain upon the involved tooth is to be masticated; only soft foods are permitted.

If the teeth are very loose, warm beeswax or ordinary candle wax placed around the crowns of the involved teeth serves very well as a temporary splint. The wax should be permitted to harden in place, with the patient biting his teeth together while the wax is setting, to accommodate the bite after the wax has hardened.

19
dislocations and joint injuries

Knee, shoulder, and ankle injuries are a prominent feature of modern-day athletic activities. Damage to the hip joint is a special hazard of old age. At any age, however, joint injuries may be serious and disabling for weeks or months or even permanently. Dislocations are shortly followed by muscle spasms, so that knowledge by the individual or the first aider that permits a return to normal position before such contractures develop can save much pain and discomfort as well as promote more rapid healing.

Damage to cartilage and other tissues of the knee commonly occurs in injuries to this structure. So commonplace are joint injuries that it is very important that the first aider understands their nature and their immediate handling.

dislocation of the shoulder

Relovszky, Kazar and E. Relovszky. "Prognosis of Primary Dislocation of the Shoulder," Acta Orthopaedica Scandinavica, 40: 216-224, Fasc. 2, 1969.

Two orthopedists from the Central Out-patient Department of the Injured in Budapest report on the medical and surgical experience in that department with 1,044 shoulder dislocations, which occurred in 966 different patients. Of the affected persons 224 had recurrent dislocations.

In this study 760 persons with a first dislocation of the shoulder were studied. *From the age of 50 years and upwards the number of shoulder dislocations was twice that of persons under the age of 50.* Below the age of 50 years dislocations were three times as frequent in men as in women, but among elderly women there were more dislocations than among the men.

Approximately 21 per cent of the patients in this research were treated because of a recurrent dislocation. One-half of the patients below the age of 20 years who had a shoulder dislocation were found to suffer from a recurrent dislocation. *For the age group 20 to 29 years, every third victim was found to have a recurrent dislocation* of the shoulder. Shoulder dislocations in the young are much more apt to be followed by similar injuries as compared to dislocations which occur for the first time in persons over the age of 50 years.

The frequency of dislocations after an initial injury is strongly related to the length of time the shoulder is immobilized after the first dislocation. Every 6th patient experienced a recurrent dislocation when the shoulder was immobilized for 3 to 7 days. However, if the shoulder was immobilized for eight to 14 days the number of recurrent dislocations was only about one-third that of fewer days of treatment.

Limitation of movement of the shoulder after a dislocation occurs mostly among the persons over the age of 50 years. Only 2 per cent of those under the age of 30 years had significant limitation, but 14 per cent of those between the ages of 31 to 50, and 37 per cent of those over the age of 50 had significant limitation of shoulder movement.

The authors agree with those authorities who believe that young persons should have a shoulder immobilized for at least 3 weeks after a dislocation in order to reduce the likelihood of a recurrent dislocation. Over the age of 50 years, however, a shorter time is advised because of the possibility of reduction in shoulder movement.

shoulder injuries

Drill, Frederick E. "Injuries of the Shoulder in Athletics," Minnesota Medicine, 48: 1665-1667, (No. 12), December 1965.

A physician of Minneapolis, Minnesota, observes that shoulder injuries do not occur often in sports, and that rehabilitation or return to normal does not take as long as when the injury occurs to the weight-bearing joints.

There are four injuries that involve the shoulder joint in athletics in terms of most frequent occurrence. These four injuries are: 1) separation of the sternum and clavicle; 2) a forward or anterior dislocation of the head of the humerus (upper arm); 3) separation or dislocation of the acromioclavicular joint, and 4) fracture of the clavicle.

Three of these problems involve only the soft tissues of the joint and with proper treatment the athlete usually can be expected to return to competition within three to six weeks from the date of the injury. The fourth type of shoulder injury, the fracture of the clavicle, can be expected to heal with a firm union of the broken parts, in about eight to 10 weeks after the injury.

The diagnosis of a shoulder injury requires that the athlete be undressed to the waist. The first step in the examination involves a visual observation to see if there is an asymmetrical contour between the two shoulders. A focus on the specific site of damage is assisted if there is evidence of bruise or abrasion. Palpation (pressure with the fingers) can bring out evidence of tenderness. *X-rays are mandatory for a full evaluation of potential damage.*

If there has been a dislocation of the joint with a spontaneous reduction, treatment with a sling or swath (a soft binding or bandage) for about three weeks is advisable. If it is necessary for the physician to reduce the dislocation under anesthesia in order to avoid further injury to soft tissues, then an x-ray after the reduction is advisable. Heavy sedation may be necessary, but straight traction on the arm is usually successful in achieving the reduction.

Some surgeons believe that open reduction (surgical opening of the shoulder) and internal fixation is advisable in both a separation or a dislocation of a shoulder joint in an athlete. Most agree that complete dislocation in an athlete demands open reduction and some type of internal fixation for six weeks. Patients who do not have proper treatment for a shoulder injury may have a rather ugly deformity, may lose strength in the shoulder and may suffer an especial loss of strength whenever the victim works with the arm above the horizontal.

self-reduction of a dislocated shoulder

Gage, E. Lyle, "Self-Reduction of Dislocated Shoulders," *West Virginia Medical Journal*, 53: 74-75 (No. 2), February 1957.

E. Lyle Gage, M.D., of Bluefield, West Virginia, observes that following the dislocation of a shoulder there is usually a period of a few minutes before the muscles of the shoulder go into spasm or before swelling begins. Reduction of the dislocation during this time is much easier than it is later when the swelling and muscle spasm are present.

Dr. Gage has himself suffered some dislocations of the left shoulder which he was able to reduce successfully without assistance from others. He reports that the method used in reducing these dislocations was as follows:

(1) The assumption of a sitting-down position.

(2) Grasping of the wrist of the dislocated arm firmly.

(3) Flexing of the leg and thigh on the side of the dislocation and slipping the joined wrists over the knee, leaning as far forward as possible.

(4) Slowly straightening the back, the thigh extended, and pushing of the knee against the wrists, exerting a pull on the arm of the dislocated side. As this movement is carried out, a tendency for the shoulder muscles to relax can be noted, then a slight "bump" at the shoulder will occur and this is followed by restored movement of the arm.

Dr. Gage reports that he reduced three dislocations of his arm within one or two minutes of the time of their occurrence, and not for several minutes after reduction was there any tightening or spasm of the muscles of the shoulder girdle. Although self-reduction in this manner may not be successful in severe cases, Dr. Gage believes it is worth a trial in an emergency.

soft tissue injuries of the knee

Drill, Frederick E. "*Athletic Injuries—Evaluation and Immediate Treatment of Soft Tissue Knee Injuries Sustained in Athletics, Minnesota Medicine, 48: 1359-62, (No. 10), October 1965. Special Issue.*

A physician of Minneapolis, Minnesota, who participated in a symposium on athletic injuries sponsored by the Minnesota Committee on Trauma of the American College of Surgeons says that *of all the joints, the knee is probably the most vulnerable to athletic* injury.

Contusion, torsion, and angulatory strain are the forces which result in injury to the knee joint. Pain and swelling (effusion) are undoubtedly the most frequent symptom and sign of knee-joint trouble; and it is usually secondary to contusion, twisting, or forced angulation.

The reaction of the athlete to his injury immediately after it has happened is often an elucidation sign as to how seriously he has been hurt. If he has full range of motion of the knee and can bear weight without persistent pain, chances are that his recovery will be rapid without residual disability. On the other hand, if the knee is locked or unstable, or if the pain is "unbearable," the athlete may be in for a long period of rehabilitation, including possible surgery, with a high probability of permanent disability.

Physical examination of the knee at the scene of the injury should include the testing of the lateral stability, both with the knee fully extended and with the knee flexed 30 degrees. Instability with the knee in full extension indicates rupture of at least one of the cruciate ligaments as well as the collateral ligament involved; instability only at 30 degrees indicates rupture of the collateral ligament in question.

A locked knee suggests strongly the possibility of a torn meniscus. The medial meniscus is much more apt to be injured than the lateral.

If a severe injury to any of the ligaments or to either of the menisci has occurred, bleeding into the joint and swelling usually follow immediately. *The quicker a bulky pressure dressing is applied, the less bleeding and effusion there will be.* Aspiration of the joint is indicated both as a diagnostic aid and as a way of relieving discomfort; it should be done under strictly aseptic technique. If there is bleeding into the joint, a tear of ligament or meniscus has most probably occurred. If there are fat globules in the aspirate, a fracture has most probably been sustained. Decreasing the intra-articular pressure definitely affords relief of pain. Pressure dressing, elevation, and ice packing are deterrents to reaccumulation of blood and joint fluid. Should bleeding into the joint recur multiple aspirations are warranted in order to avoid the complications of protracted resorption of the blood, which leads to synovial reaction, formation of fibrin deposits, and adhesions.

In the case where a sprain has occurred and there is a possibility of internal derangement a cylinder cast for 2 to 3 weeks is indicated. This will allow soft-tissue healing to take place with the knee immobilized. and the patient will be comfortable. He may bear full weight without fear of the knee hurting or buckling.

If the patient has either a locked knee or rupture of ligaments, consultation concerning early surgical repair is certainly indicated.

An athlete should not be allowed to return to participation until there is no longer any swelling. He may be able to participate, but he will in most instances do damage to his knee if he engages in athletic activity while there is still effusion present. Rehabilitation consists of isometric progressive resistance exercises of the quadriceps, guarded and progressive weight bearing with crutches, and active range of motion exercises until full range of motion is achieved. The quadri ceps of the injured knee should be at least as strong as — and preferable stronger than — those of the normal knee. If ligaments have been severely strained or torn, the knee should probably be protected with criss-cross taping during future competition.

ankle injuries

Drill, Frederick. "Management of Ankle Injuries Sustained in Sports," Minnesota Medicine, 48: 1173-74, (No. 9), September 1965.

A physician of Minneapolis, Minnesota, participating in a conference on fractures and injuries associated with sports, states that with an athlete who has suffered any injury to the ankle, *it is best to bring the athlete to the sidelines without permitting him to bear any weight on the injured extremity.*

Once on the sidelines, the shoe and any tape should be removed and a careful examination made of the injured ankle. It is well to make frequent comparisons with the normal ankle, in respect to the relative ranges of motion and stability of the various ligaments.

Ankle injuries can be classified into any one of four categories of severity, ranging from the least degree of injury to a complete rupture. A grade 1 sprain indicates the least degree of injury. A grade 2 sprain, if properly treated with a cooperative patient, can be healed in about eight days after the injury and the athlete may be permitted to return to full competition. Only in the case of minor injuries (grade one), where there is full range of motion of the ankle, good stability, and no significant pain when stress is placed upon the various ligaments, should the team physician permit the athlete to return immediately to the game. If there is evidence of rupture of a blood vessel, or swelling due to blood, then a grade 2, 3 or 4 sprain must be suspected and the player must be prohibited from any further immediate participation on the day of injury.

Minor, or grade 1 sprains, require rewrapping of the ankle if the athlete is to return immediately to the game. After the game the foot should be elevated and the ankle packed in ice for 24 hours. After this period of time whirlpool treatment and active exercises will speed complete recovery.

Sprains of grade 2 or 3 variety call for immediate exclusion from the game, pressure dressing, ice-packing, elevation of the ankle, and rest. For weight-bearing the ankle should be supported with tape-strapping or a short-leg walking cast. The patient should be kept on crutches with partial weight bearing until he can walk without pain or limp. This phase of the treatment may require from seven to 21 days.

In severe injuries involving fractures or dislocations there is usually little pain for about 30 minutes, unless the tibial nerve has been stretched. Hemorrhage and swelling will occur first. During this period of time the foot and ankle can be manipulated back to normal alignment. Grade 4 sprains involve fractures; x-rays are necessary. A cast for this severe form of ankle sprain should be left in place for six weeks without weight bearing. Post-cast x-rays should be taken.

20
unconsciousness

Loss of consciousness can come from many different physical causes that may reflect changes in the normal physiology of the body, biochemical alterations due to disease or temporary conditions, lack of oxygen due to near-drowning or other causes, simple shifts in circulation that permit a pooling of blood in certain parts of the body, head injuries or other direct damage, psychological stresses, or many other causes, almost without limit.

So far as the first aider is concerned it cannot be expected that he can with certainty identify the cause of unconsciousness, but he can and should swiftly ascertain if the heart has stopped or if breathing has been impaired, for these are conditions that he can do something about that may save the life of the person involved.

fainting

Williams, Robert L., and Peter D. Allen. "Loss of Consciousness," Aerospace Medicine, 33: 545-551, (No. 5), May, 1962.

A flight surgeon and an assistant from the College of Medicine of the University of Florida at Gainesville says the conscious state is one in which the individual is alert, receptive and responsive to external and internal stimuli. At the other end of the spectrum is the phenomenon described as unconsciousness. There are varying degrees of "unconsciousness," but in general it may be described as a gross or major disturbance; a state in which the human organism is not alert to external or internal stimuli; is probably minimally, if at all, receptive to stimuli; and responds poorly, if at all.

The authors conducted a survey of a large college population to determine the incidence of loss of consciousness, and to determine what major "causes" are associated with episodes of loss of consciousness. As a second phase of the study, electroencephalograms were performed on a sample of the population surveyed and the recordings interpreted as normal or abnormal.

Eight hundred and seventy-one persons were questioned: 95 women and 776 men with an average age of 21.1 years. The major causes of loss of consciousness presented to each subject included episodes of severe pain, postural change, exertion, receiving medications or injections (not anesthetics), infections, trauma to the head, loss of or donation of blood, intake of alcohol, accidental breathing of poisonous or unpleasant fumes, and emotional experiences.

Of the 871 students surveyed, 47.1 per cent had experienced at least one episode of loss of consciousness. Of the episodes, 74.3 per cent were caused by trauma to the head, intake of alcohol, pain, and postural change, in that order. These same four stimuli accounted for 75 per cent of the episodes experienced by the males in the population, whereas pain, trauma to the head, postural change and infections accounted for 70.5 per cent of the episodes experienced by the females in the group.

Trauma to the head was experienced by 55.4 per cent of the subjects, thus not only causing the greatest number of episodes, but also being experienced by the greatest number of people. Pain was the most common stimulus for the females, and trauma to the head for the males.

The electroencephalographic studies on a sample of the population revealed no correlation between the incidence of EEG abnormalities and the incidence of loss of consciousness.

This survey shows that the incidence of loss of consciousness in a healthy population is much higher than others have assumed.

fainting spells

Dermksian, George, and Lawrence E. Lamb. "Syncope in a Population of Healthy Young Adults," Journal of the American Medical Association, 168: 1200-07, (No. 9), Nov. 1, 1958.

Two physicians of the School of Aviation Medicine, Randolph Air Force Base, Texas, report a study of 82 persons who had 113 fainting episodes. All of the 82 persons were apparently healthy members of the Air Force flying personnel.

According to these physicians, *fainting is a common, everyday occurence,* often due to more than a single cause. One investigator found that nearly 16 per cent of a group of 300 healthy, young college males had fainting episodes. In this study, approximately 3,000 questionnaires were obtained from air force personnel of an average age of 29 years, to ascertain the frequency of fainting spells. It was found that 7 per cent had experienced what could be diagnosed as true fainting spells.

The mechanisms resulting in fainting can be classified into six general categories, as follows: 1) inadequate return of blood to the left heart; 2) ineffective pumping action of the heart; 3) a change in routing of the blood flow due to loss of arteriolar tone; 4) abnormalities in the contents of the circulating blood; 5) inadequate circulating blood volume and 6) local disorders of the central nervous system. More than one mechanism may be involved in a single fainting spell.

Disturbances of cardiac rhythm are a major factor in causing inefficient pumping action of the heart. The pulmonary stretch reflex (which is stimulated by breath-holding and pressure breathing) is frequently involved in causing a disturbance of cardiac rhythm. The stretch reflex may be due to some unexplained deaths in underwater swimming. The stretch may be of particular importance in all occupations involving pressure breathing, altitude exposure, and other forms of respiratory stimulation. The stretch reflex may play a significant role in producing distrubances of cardiac rhythm and cardiac arrest during artificial respiration. The vagal response to the stretch reflex is abolished by atropine, and this knowledge may have applications in both industry and medicine.

Fainting spells occurred in this group under the following circumstances: unexplained, while playing cards; flying at 8,000 feet; seated after lack of food, lack of sleep and exertion; after lack of sleep while shaving; on rising from a chair; back pain; on getting out of bed; on drinking alcohol; during dental procedures; while watching his child have a nosebleed; on the sight of blood; while standing at a racetrack; on falling out of bed; on straightening up after bending over;

on hyperventilating; on straining at stool; on having a gastrointestinal infection; on urinating; on standing in line for a physical examination; on seeing a dog hit by a car; while coughing; after vomiting; while standing at attention in the sun; after turning in his seat at 31,000 feet altitude; while mowing the lawn, and so on. Alcohol ingestion was mentioned frequently as being associated with fainting.

multiple causes of unconsciousness

Thomas M. Marshall, "Management of the Unconscious Patient," Journal of the Kentucky State Medical Association, 54: 157-61 (No. 2), February 1956.

Thomas M. Marshall, M.D., of Louisville, Kentucky, observes that *the unconscious patient presents an emergency problem of great importance.* In his discussion of the medical aspects of treatment and diagnosis, Dr. Marshall also stresses the importance of adequate first aid measures. The establishment and maintenance of an adequate airway takes precedence over all other problems. All too often the comatose patient is in the supine position when found. This position provides conditions extremely unfavorable to proper ventilation. Nasal and oral secretions, vomitus, blood, and a relaxed tongue can readily gravitate into the throat. This obstruction can easily be prevented by placing the patient on his side or in the Schaefer resuscitation posture.

An accurate history provided by a member of the patient's family, a friend, the police, or an onlooker will often make the diagnosis simple. A story of injury, previous strokes, hypertension, suicide attempts, drug or alcoholic ingestion, recent infection, headaches and vomiting, convulsions, known diabetes, or pregnancy often provides the necessary background to the physician for a proper diagnosis. The place where the patient is found in his unconscious state often provides valuable information.

Causes of unconsciousness encompass almost the entire field of medicine. Dr. Marshall uses the word COMA-PIC (coma-picture) as a means of recalling leading factors that may be involved in unconsciousness. In the word COMA-PIC, the "C" stands for cerebral factor; "O" for opium and other drugs, chemicals, and metallic toxins; "M" for metabolic factors; "A" for anemic factors; "P" for psychogenie disturbances; "I" for infectious agents; and "C" for cardiovascular factors.

Cerebral factors include injury, vascular accidents such as hemorrhage or blood clots in the brain, brain tumors, degenerative diseases, and post-convulsive stupor. Opium and its numerous derivatives represent the drug intoxications. Other commonly-encountered agents include alcohol, barbiturates, bromides, carbon monoxides, and lead. Alcoholism is a factor *in almost three out of five cases of unconsciousness.*

Metabolic factors that may be related to unconsciousness include diabetes mellitus, low blood sugar, underactive thyroid, heat exhaustion, sun-stroke, and so on. Anemic factors include hemorrhages, the anemias, and the leukemias. Psychogenic disturbances include malingering psycho-neuroses and psychoses. The infectious agents include pneumonia, meningitis, influenza, tetanus, and other diseases. Cardiovascular factors include coronary occlusions and other heart and circulatory conditions, including cardiac arrest.

unconscious diabetic patient

Martin, Marguerite M. *"The Unconscious Diabetic Patient," American Journal of Nursing, 61: 92-94, (No. 11), November 1961.*

A nurse of St. Joseph's Hospital, Willimantic, Connecticut says that when an individual known to have diabetes is found in an unconscious state, one first considers that he has one of the two diabetic emergencies: diabetic coma or insulin reaction. Diabetic coma is a serious complication of the disease. Insulin reaction is a possible side effect of insulin therapy. To tell the difference between the two states occasionally proves difficult, although they are medical opposites.

It should be remembered that the diabetic patient is not immune to other medical emergencies, and these must also be considered. Some of the more common possibilities are cerebral hemorrhage, uremia, meningitis, and brain injury or tumor.

The patient's history is very important in differentiating diabetic coma, insulin reaction, and the before-mentioned conditions. A relative of the unconscious patient can often be very helpful. Also, the modern hospital laboratory makes possible a rapid and accurate diagnosis. Insulin should never be administered to an unconscious diabetic person until the reason for loss of consciousness has been established.

The following table lists the different symptoms and characteristics of both states:

	Diabetic Coma	*Insulin Reaction*
Onset	Slow-days	Sudden minutes or hours
Food	Too much	Too little
Insulin	Too little	Too much
Presence of infection	Frequent	None
Thirst	Extreme	Absent
Hunger	Absent	Frequent
Vomiting	Common	Seldom
Pain in abdomen	Frequent	Absent
Fever	Absent, except with infection	Absent
Skin	Dry	Moist
Tremor	Absent	Frequent
Vision	Dim	Double
Eyeballs	Soft	Normal
Appearance	Florid—extremely ill	Pale weak faint
Respiration	Air-hunger	Normal
Blood pressure	Tends to fall	Tends to rise
Mental state	Restless—distressed	Apathetic irritable hysterical
Unconsciousness	Gradually approaches	May intervene suddenly
Specific treatment	Insulin—fluid—salt	Carbohydrate
Response to treatment	Gradual—hours	Quick minutes

The primary cause of diabetic coma is insulin deficiency. When there is a lack of insulin—either natural or omission of injected insulin—the body is unable to utilize glucose to the full extent of its metabolic needs for enrgy. The body then has to fall back on proteins and particularly fat for its caloric requirements. When this occurs, an over-stimulation of fat metabolism occurs. Fatty acids are converted into ketone bodies in the liver. These ketone bodies are toxic when produced faster than the body's capacity to use them for energy needs. In diabetic coma, ketone bodies accumulate in the blood and urine in large quantities and a toxic complication exists.

In the unknown diabetic person, the disorder may go undetected until a state of acidosis or coma develops. In the known diabetic person, acidosis and coma are frequently the result of neglect or ignorance. The onset and symptoms of diabetic coma are described in the table on the previous page.

Insulin shock, the second diabetic emergency, results when the blood sugar level drops from a normal, or above normal, level to a sub-normal one, becuase of too much insulin. It does not necessarily mean that too much insulin was injected. It may indicate that, for one reason or another, the body needed less insulin at that time. One can summarize by saying that insulin reaction results from too much insulin, too little food, or exercise poorly planned.

Diabetes in some individuals, particularly children and young adults, is more unstable than in some others, and these diabetic persons are particularly prone to insulin reactions.

Insulin reactions which are treated promptly are over quickly. All diabetic patients are taught how to recognize the onset of a reaction and to carry some form of carbohydrate. Fruit juice, carbonated drinks, sugar, or small candies will correct the condition quickly. The neglected, prolonged reaction—although rarely fatal—can have serious consequences. This type is most apt to occur if the diabetic patient fails to pay attention to the early warning signals, or if the onset occurs during his sleeping hours. If a patient lapses into unconsciousness because of insulin reaction, the best treatment is the intravenous administration of 50 per cent glucose solution. He should regain consciousness within a few minutes.

Diabetic coma is the more serious of the two conditions, because the lack of diabetic control which it indicates can, if continued, lead eventually to disabling vascular lesions in the eyes, kidneys, heart, or extremities. Early recognition, however, usually leads to prompt and adequate treatment.

head injuries and coma

Webster, John E. "The Unconscious State in Head Injuries," Clinical Neurosurgery, 3: 202-23, Annual, 1955.

A physician observes that *whenever the head is struck it undergoes a change in velocity due to the blow.* In addition to the deformation of the skull, the change in the velocity produces pressure changes within the cranial cavity. This effect of acceleration is in addition to the forces produced by the deformation of the skull when struck. When the head is struck the area receiving the blow bends in, thus reducing the volume and increasing the pressure within the cranial cavity. In some cases, high acceleration may produce no physiological response, while in others low accelerations yield concussion or death.

Direct and indirect injuries to the head may cause the following basic mechanical effect:

(1) Compression

(2) Acceleration

(3) Deceleration

Compression, acceleration and deceleration may cause:

(1) Deformation of head and skull and compression of contents.

(2) A sudden increase in intracranial pressure.

(3) Mass movements of intracranial contents.

(4) Distortion of the skull and the outermost membrane covering the brain.

(5) Shearing off a portion of head without necessarily producing increased intracranial pressure.

(6) Shearing and tearing with intense increased intracranial pressure.

Experiments have shown that in blunt injuries of the head, where major distortion of the skull and its contents does not take place, and where extensive failure of bond is not present, the effects of the blow are due primarily to a sudden increase in intracranial pressure at the time of impact. This increase of pressure may be as much as 15 to 100 pounds per square inch. These changes in pressure are caused by the deformation of the skull and the acceleration or deceleration of the head due to the impact. The area which receives the most injury under these circumstances appears to be the neural tissue of the brain stem.

Brain concussion occurs as a result of brain stem injury. It is associated with *unconsciousness, pallor, and a shock-like state.* The brain stem involvement may be of varying degrees, involving both reversible and irreversible damage. A reversible state may result in complete recovery: the irreversible in unconsciousness with ultimate death.

coma mechanisms

Fazekas, Joseph F., and Alice N. Bessman. "Coma Mechanisms," American Journal of Medicine, 15: 804-12, (No. 6), December 1953.

Joseph F. Fazekas, M.D., and Alice N. Bessman, M.D., of Washington, D.C., report that *many disorders of the brain result from metabolic disturbances within the central nervous system.* If energy deprivation is of sufficient magnitude and duration, regardless of cause, coma and possibly irreversible damage may result.

Normal functioning of the brain depends upon reactions between an adequate supply of energy and oxygen. Glucose is the principal source of energy, although the brain can also oxidize certain amino acids as well as fatty acids which are synthesized within the cerebral cells. The brain is highly dependent for its supply of energy on the glucose delivered to it via the circulation. Any marked reduction in the delivery of glucose to the brain will result in impairment of function and if this impairment lasts long enough will result in coma. An insufficiency of oxygen will also produce the same result. Enzymes act as catalysts in the reactions between glucose and oxygen. Any inhibition or the lack of essential enzymes for the breakdown of glucose will, therefore, also result in metabolic disturbances of the brain.

In coma from diabetes, liver disease, alcoholism, barbiturates, pernicious anemia, and other conditions there is a major disturbance of the enzymes that are necessary for the use of energy and oxygen by the tissues of the brain. In strangulation, heart failure, and cerebral arteriosclerosis, oxygen deficiency may be a major cause of coma. A marked deficiency in blood sugar may result in coma even when the enzyme system is undisturbed and there is adequate oxygen.

Some of the cerebral enzymes are hexokinase, pyruvic oxidase, and cytochrome oxidase.

Comas associated with a virus infection, and possibly the degenerative diseases of the central nervous system, may be due primarily to a destruction or inactivation of enzymes.

The adult brain cannot function for even short periods of time in the absence of oxygen but must be constantly supplied with it to meet its metabolic requirements. Oxygen deprivation from whatever cause, for even short periods of time, results in structural and functional changes in the central nervous system.

The effects of oxygen deprivation and low blood sugar on the central nervous system are clinically and pathologically the same.

unconsciousness from underwater swimming

Craig, Albert B. Jr., "Underwater Swimming and Loss of Consciousness," The Journal of the American Medical Association, 176: 87-90, (No. 4), April 29, 1961.

A physician of the Department of Physiology of the University of Rochester School of Medicine and Dentistry reports that in recent years it has been possible to obtain valuable information from swimmers who have trod the fine line between life and death in underwater swimming. Eight such swimmers, all of whom were attempting to swim relatively long distances under water, were interviewed by this physician. One of the case studies is cited below:

"A good swimmer, age 18, decided to repeat a previous performance he had achieved by swimming under water for three laps of a 75-ft. pool, *i.e.*, 225 ft. He hyperventilated for about one minute, at which time he was dizzy. A significant urge to breathe was not apparent until the beginning of the third lap, when he reminded himself that his goal was 225 ft.

He did not remember swimming most of the third lap. When he reached the end, a fellow student, who was watching the swim specifically, reported that the subject surfaced but that he failed to raise his head. He began to cough and gasp, but regained consciousness in two or three breaths, after his head was held above the surface. The subject did not recall any aftereffects other than being slightly tired."

All of the survivors studied were considered good swimmers and experienced at underwater swimming. There were other common factors. They all did deep breathing before going under the surface. Seven of the eight had some goal in mind or were in competition with others. The swimmer usually noted the urge to breathe but had little or no warning that he was going to "pass out." Some of the swimmers continued to make coordinated movements and one even executed a turn at the end of the pool beyond the point of remembrance. Observers of these swimmers did not suspect that a problem existed until final collapse occurred.

These events have been investigated by means of experiments to explain why a person might lose consciousness while swimming underwater. It was found that hyperventilation (deep breathing) preceding breath-holding and exercise may delay the sensation of the urge to breathe. Before the partial pressure of carbon dioxide increases significantly, the oxygen may decrease to a degree incompatible with high-level cerebral function.

Prevention of this type of accident is the logical answer to the problem, for underwater swimming is quite safe under certain circumstances and may be a useful skill to know. Prolonged or severe hyperventilation should be discouraged before attempting the underwater swim, and the urge to breathe, when felt, should not be ignored for long.

unconsciousness from lack of oxygen

Flagg, Paluel J. "Asphyxia—Consciousness Will Save Life," GP, VIII: 41-44, (No. 2), August, 1953.

A physician of New York City says there are many different causes of asphyxia, but that a common overall treatment can rescue the victim in each condition.

Asphyxia is loss of consciousness as a result of too little oxygen; it may lead to death if treatment is not begun at once. Asphyxia may be due to many different causes, such as smothering, suffocation, drowning, smoke inhalation, concealed hemorrhage, foreign-body obstruction, poisoning from drugs or alcohol, electrocution, carbon monoxide poisoning, and many others. But the effect on the body is the same in each case: hypoxia (reduction of oxygen supply to the tissues). The treatment, once the cause is removed, is identical. It involves getting more oxygen into the blood stream.

Each year in the United States over 50,000 deaths occur from asphyxia. This is almost twice as many deaths as those occurring from automobile accidents. *Many of these deaths might be prevented with a little greater knowledge of resuscitation methods and with more immediate action.*

The hazard of asphyxia is gravest at birth. Each year 35,000 deaths at birth are charged to hypoxia. The other 15,000 result from the causes mentioned above.

While death from hypoxia claims at least 50,000 lives each year, the late, non-fatal effects are becoming generally recognized. Exposure to hypoxia may result in profound disturbances to the nervous systems of those who survive. Brain tissue is the first to suffer damage from lack of oxygen. Hypoxia is one of the accepted causes of cerebral palsy. Mental defects of children are often traced to protracted hypoxia at birth. It also accounts for many late mental defects; adults who survive protracted asphyxia may live a mere vegetative existence. Preventive efforts might well reduce the number of cases of asphyxia, especially at birth.

Instant diagnosis and immediate action are imperative in the treatment of asphyxia. When a physician is available, he should instantly appraise the degree of asphyxia, for there are different stages. Each stage is the result of changes which constitute specific indications for treatment. The stages are depression, spasticity, and flaccidity. *The lay rescuer, however, should be concerned with two facts: (1) cessation of breathing indicates a grave emergency, and (2) mouth-to-mouth resuscitation should be started immediately* and kept up until a physician arrives and the victim is hospitalized.

21
gunshot and missile wounds

Injuries caused by gunshot may differ to an extraordinary extent because of the part of the body that may be entered by the missile, by its velocity, by its direction and by still other factors. Even the term "gunshot" has become more complicated because of the advent of modern weapons such as mines, shrapnel, missiles and other sources of injury to which combat personnel in particular may be exposed. However, much similarity exists between wounds caused by these substances. One of the important factors is the damage caused by the formation of a cavity in the body in the path of the bullet or other metal which stretches, tears, or otherwise damages nearby tissue even though it is not in the immediate path of the bullet.

All gunshot wounds represent a surgical emergency and exploration of the body in the injured area is a necessity for detection of damaged blood vessels and other tissues that might not be otherwise found. Obviously the immediate role of the first aider in gunshot cases is that of controlling as much as possible the always-present bleeding, sustaining breathing, and getting the victim to a physician or surgeon at a hospital as quickly as possible.

human missile wounds

Finck, Pierre A. "A Research Concept for the Interpretation of Human Missile Wounds by the Pathologist," Military Medicine, 135: 912-913, (No. 10), October 1970.

The Chief of the Wound Ballistics Pathology Branch of the Armed Forces Institute of Pathology in Washington, D.C., in making recommendations regarding the types of information that pathologists should study when wounds are caused by missiles such as bullets, also calls attention to certain facts about definitions regarding gunshot wounds.

Research that has given knowledge on the "temporary cavity" has contributed immensely to the understanding of the mechanism of wounding. *The temporary cavity within the tissue lasts only a few thousandths of a second, but during this brief period of time it creates pressures that are often in excess of 1,000 pounds per inch.* This phenomenon, which is greater as the velocity of the projectile increases, helps to explain damage or disturbance of function in tissues at a distance from the missile path or track.

In a penetrating wound the anatomy of the body shows an entry of the bullet or other missile, but does not show an exit. In a perforating wound (through-and-through) the anatomy of the body shows both an entry and exit point. Sometimes a projectile breaks up into fragments, some of which may be retained in the body, but may sometimes cause a wound of exit as it leaves the body. Thus, an exit wound may be caused by the primary missile or it may be caused by a secondary missile that has been set into motion by the first. The latter kind of injury is called a perforating wound with retention of fragments.

High velocity wounds (caused by missiles travelling at least 2,500 feet per second) do not necessarily result in perforation. Some bullets of high velocity often break up within the human body and do not always produce a wound of exit. Fragments of a certain hand grenade, for example, have a velocity of about 5,000 feet per second, but most of the fragments are retained in the body.

missile wounds of the blood vessels

Amato, Joseph J., Lawrence J. Billy, Ronald P. Gruber, Noel S. Lawson and Norman M. Rich. "Vascular Injuries. An Experimental Study of High and Low Velocity Missile Wounds," Archives of Surgery, 101: 167-174, (No. 2), August 1970.

Five military physicians report on the mechanism of injury to blood vessels that may occur from missiles of various masses and velocities. Experimental studies by the group involving the use of high-speed photography have established that significant damage to arteries may be caused by the crushing effect in the formation of a temporary cavity as the bullet or missile penetrates tissue.

The temporary cavity is explained by the sudden release of energy that is directly proportional to the mass and velocity of the bullet. Arteries not injured by a bullet may be literally torn apart by the release of energy in the temporary cavity that follows the bullet. Experimental studies have shown that in animals the damage to blood vessels is proportional to their nearness to the center of the cavity and injuries become less significant as the vessel lies further from the center of the temporary cavity.

Low-velocity missiles are apt to push blood vessels ahead slightly before penetration. High-velocity missiles neatly shear the wall of the artery, but an "explosive effect" of the temporary cavity created by the bullet causes "blunt" injuries in a crushing manner. Microscopic changes in the walls of arteries have been found in all three layers and at all velocities. The microscopic damages that were found included *disruption of tissues of the arteries, herniation, bleeding and multiple small blood clots.* These mechanical injuries extended to approximately eight inches or more in most of the arteries examined.

High-speed photography revealed that missiles could pass by an artery without damaging it or even moving it, but then the vessel would be violently disrupted by the temporary cavity.

The first effect of a high velocity missile involves the transference of energy at impact with tissue, in a so-called "blowing out" effect that causes sudden collapse or bursting inward of soft tissue. A second effect is thermal in nature, because most missiles are hot when they penetrate soft tissue. Finally, most missiles are wobbling when they hit and the tumbling or shimmy effect may be involved in the energy transference. Another effect is known as the bounce phenomenon. Bullets do not always penetrate; they sometimes hit hard tissues, such as a rib, vertebra, or other bone and may bounce around in the body cavities and cause a great deal of havoc to various tissues and organs.

penetrating wounds of the great arteries of the chest

Panagiotis, N. Symbas, Jagjit S. Sehdeva, Osler A. Abbott, Charles R. Hatcher, Jr. and William D. Logan, Jr. "Penetrating Wounds of the Thoracic Aorta and Great Arteries," Southern Medical Journal, 63: 853-857, (No. 7), July 1970.

Five physicians of Emory University School of Medicine in Atlanta, Georgia, report that *a penetrating or lacerating injury to the great blood vessels of the chest is usually fatal.* A bullet or stab wound affecting these vessels usually causes such a loss of blood that the victim bleeds to death before a medical facility can be reached to render proper care. Even a great number of such injured patients who arrive alive at an emergency clinic will perish before adequate care can be provided.

Even with the most rapid transportation to a hospital, the victim is seldom able to be saved by surgery. In a patient who does survive long enough to be helped by surgical correction, there has usually been an interruption of the bleeding process because of sealing of the damaged vessel by a clot or adjoining tissues.

The proper care of the patient with penetrating wounds of the great blood vessels calls for rapid and vigorous measures. Adequate ventilation (breathing) must be established, routes for the rapid administration of massive amounts of blood or blood volume expanders must be instituted, blood and air must be evacuated from the chest cavity, and the rapid determination of any injury to body organs must be made. These measures, of course, must be taken by the surgeon and it should be apparent that patients with massive bleeding must be operated upon immediately.

index

Abdominal injuries, 144-147, 150-153, 251-252
Allergic reactions, 25-27, 72-75, 189-192
Ambulances, 10-11
Amphetamine overdosage, 109
Anaphylactic shock, 72-75, 189-192
Animal bites, 204-206
Ankle injuries, 13, 230-232
Arteries, wounds to, 3, 47-58, 248-250
Artificial respiration, 30-41, 118
Aspirin poisoning, 129-130, 134-135
Assessment of accident situations, 5-6
Athletes, sudden deaths of, 23-25

Bad trips, 110, 112-114
Barbiturate overdosage, 110-111
Bee sting, 72-75, 189-192
Bites, 190-206
Black Widow spider bite, 193-196
Bleeding, 2-3, 7, 9, 53-66, 69-72 153, 249-250
Blood in the urine, 153
Brain hemorrhage, signs of, 56-57, 86
Breath-holding spells, 38-39

Breathing, 2-3, 9, 22-23, 29-49, 78, 80, 82, 118
Brief psychotherapy, 96-99
Broken eardrums, 93-94
Brown Spider bites, 192-193
Burns, 155-170
Burns, cold treatment of, 157-158
Cardiac emergencies, 15-27, 33, 46, 235
Cardiac massage, 18-23, 46
Cardiac rhythm, disturbances of, 17, 25-27, 235
Chest injury, 149-150, 250
Chilblains, 182
Child abuse, 107-108
Choking, 37-38
Cloth burns, 156-157
Clotting process, 53-54
Coagulation, 53-54
Cold injuries, 179-188
Cold treatment of injuries, 12-13, 157-158
Coma, 237-242
Concussion, 87-88
Corrosives, 136-137
Cortisone, 11-12

Dental injuries, 91, 219-223
Desensitization treatment, 74-75
Detachment of retina, 209-211
Diabetic coma, 237-240
Dilated pupil, 78, 80-81
Dislocations, 225-232

Dog bites, 204-206
Drowning, 33-37, 43-51, 242-244
Drug reactions, 109-124, 207-208
Drugs, bad trips, 110, 112-114

Eardrums, broken, 93-94
Electrical injuries, 33, 163-170.
Electrical burns of the mouth, 163-164
Emergency psychotherapy, 96-99
Epilepsy, 83, 88
Epistaxis, 61-64
Eve method, 34-36
External cardiac massage, 18-23, 46
Eye burns, 215-217
Eye, foreign body in the, 211-213
Eye injuries, 211-218

Facial burns, 159-161
Facial injuries, 89-92, 159-160
Fainting, 233-236
Fever, 78, 172, 174, 177
Fibrillation, 25-26
Food sensitivity, 25-27
Foreign bodies in the eye, 211-213
Fractures, 3, 8, 10, 13, 21-22
Frostbite, 179-180, 182-188

Gunshot wounds, 247-250

Hallucinogen reactions, 110

Head injuries, 3, 54-57, 77-94, 240-241
Hearing, loss of, 93-94
Heart attacks, 15-27, 66
Heart failure, 46
Heat cramps, 173, 176
Heat exhaustion, 173, 176
Heat injuries, 171-178
Heat prostration, 173, 176
Heat stroke, 172-176
Hemorrhage, 2-3, 7, 9, 53-66, 69-72, 153, 249-250
Heroin, 117-124
Hyperbaric oxygen, 23

Immersion foot, 188
Inflammation, 11
Insecticide poisoning, 125-128
Insulin shock, 237-240
Internal injuries, 139-153, 247-252
Joint injuries, 225-232

Kerosene poisoning, 132, 134
Kidney injury, 152-153
Knee injuries, 229-230

Lead poisoning, 135-136
Lightning, deaths from, 169-170
Lysosome, 11-12

Marijuana reaction, 110
Mini-neurological examination, 81-82
Missile wounds, 247-252
Mobile heart units, 15-16
Multiple injuries, 3-4

Neck injury, 140-143
Newborn narcotic addict, 123-124
Nose, broken, 92
Nosebleed, 61-64

Opiates, 17
Oxygen, 17, 23, 29-30, 48, 67-68, 78, 178, 244-245

Pesticide poisoning, 125-128
Poisonings, 125-137
Pregnant woman, injuries to, 143-147
Principles of first aid, 1-13
Psychiatric emergencies, 95-108
Psychiatric results of injuries, 88-89
Psychiatric symptoms of children, 95-96
Psychotherapy, 96-99
Pulse rate, 80-81
Pupil, dilation of, 78-80

Rabies, 204-206
Removal of traffic victims, 6-9
Respiratory distress, 2-3, 9, 22-23, 29-49, 78, 80, 82, 118
Retina, detachment of, 209-211

Scalp injuries, 82-83
Schafer method, 32-37
Seat belts, 143-144, 147-149
Severely injured patient, 1-3
Shock, 2, 17, 60-61, 65-75
Shock, anaphylactic, 72-75
Shock lung, 67-68

Shoulder, dislocation of, 225-228
Shoulder injuries, 225-228
Skull fractures, 83, 85, 91
Snake bits, 190-192, 196-204
Solvent inhalation, 109
Spider bites, 192-196
Spinal cord injuries, 7-8, 139-143
Spleen, rupture of, 152
Splints, 8, 10, 140
Stings, reactions to, 189-192
Sudden deaths of athletes, 23-25
Suicide, potential and attempted, 100-104

Tachycardia, 26
Tear gas, 208-209
Teeth, injuries to, 91, 219-223
Temporary cavity in gunshot wounds, 247-250
Tooth extraction, bleeding from, 219-220
Tourniquet, 58-61, 74
Traffic victims, 5-11, 99-100
Tranquilizers, 110
Transportation of the injured, 3, 10-11, 139-143
Trench foot, 188
Tuberculosis, 40-41

Unconsciousness, 3, 6, 55, 77-82, 85, 141-142, 233-245
Underwater swimming, 242-244

Vapor sniffing, 109
Vision, emergencies of, 207-218

Visual complications, 87, 207-208

Windchill factor, 183-186
Wound healing, 11-12